Medicine and Literature

The doctor's companion to the classics

Volume 2

John Salinsky

D1330014

Radcliffe Medical Press
Oxford • San Francisco

Radcliffe Medical Press Ltd
18 Marcham Road
Abingdon
Oxon OX14 1AA
United Kingdom

www.radcliffe-oxford.com
The Radcliffe Medical Press electronic catalogue and online ordering facility.
Direct sales to anywhere in the world.

British Library Cataloguing in Publication Data

A catalogue record for this book is available from the British Library.

ISBN 1 85775 830 7

Typeset by Advance Typesetting Ltd, Oxfordshire
Printed and bound by TJ International Ltd, Padstow, Cornwall

Contents

Foreword

When the American poet (and novelist and storyteller and essayist) William Carlos Williams was not at his desk 'scrawling on paper', as he once put it, he was busy living the daily life of a physician – seeing patients in his Rutherford, New Jersey office, or going on home visits to the many ailing children he saw, or the grown-ups whose difficulties he also attended to. I was privileged to accompany this 'writing doctor' (as some of us called him sometimes) and to sit in his office and hear him reflect on what it meant to work at making life a bit better for his fellow human beings who were sick for one reason or another. One day, as he took to remembering particular times of trial and strain – children hurting, even dying, and their parents devastated – he turned the table round, addressed his own personal struggles as one who so relentlessly saw life's grim side, and he did so not out of 'unreflecting egoism' (as George Eliot put it in *Middlemarch*) but in an earnest, and yes humble, effort to figure out (and declare for a young physician just starting out in his professional life) what helped him keep his spirits reasonably high as a doctor, amid the melancholy that came his way all the time. A lowering of the head, a stare through a nearby window at a street he knew so well, a sigh that set the stage for the deeply felt words that followed: 'A lot of talk these days [1955] of psychology – talk of what's going on when you treat patients (in them or in you, the doc they've come to see). I read all that, and I say "sure thing" to myself; but I'll tell you, when I want to know the real rock bottom truth about what happens all the time in this doctoring life, what happens to us using our stethoscopes and our neurological hammers, and what happens to the folks who bring us their hearts and worries to be heard, their nerves to be tested, or their observer upstairs, called "the mind" to be evaluated – that's when I turn, every time, to the novelists, the playwrights, the poets, the essayists, who have given us the sights and sounds, the feel of all that goes on, minute by minute, in what we doctors call the clinical encounter: the ups and downs of hope that fades into alarm, worry, unnerving fear; and the shifts of trust, of outright distrust – so much to observe, to keep in mind, as we try to understand what it means to be a practising doctor, or a needy, vulnerable patient. What Tolstoy and Chekhov knew we need to know for ourselves, for our own sakes, as we live out our medical lives. After all, writers like those two, and others, are our lifelong teachers, advisors, friends.'

What Dr Williams asserted with evident insistence, even passion, all of us who have become physicians have reason to know, and to know inwardly with gratitude, upon meeting the pages of this carefully assembled, wonderfully telling book – a 'companion' for sure, a lasting and most helpful one, for the medical travelling that awaits us.

Robert Coles MD
Professor of Psychiatry and Medical Humanities
Harvard Medical School
November 2003

Foreword

It's odd – or is it? – how many great writers of fiction were (or planned to be) doctors. From Chekhov and Bulgakov to Somerset Maugham, Richard Gordon and Jed Mercurio – the line extends. Odd, too – or is it? – how many doctors are (or want to be) creative writers. I suspect that the medical profession has more than its expected share of novels in its collective bottom drawer, if not actually on publishers' lists.

Why should this be? At first sight you'd have thought the jobs of authorship and medicine were incompatible. Being a doctor means working out there in the world's blood and misery with the sleeves rolled up. We suppose that the writer, by contrast, inhabits a solitary and sheltered inner world, where the life of the imagination teems with no less turbulence, but silently, invisibly, evidenced only by the quiet patterns of ink upon page.

Yet both are wrestling with the same universal conundrum: how to make sense of the human condition as people – patients or characters – struggle in the relentless grip of their destiny. To be sure, author and doctor express their insights differently, the one in language, the other in action. But both professions are predicated upon a similar depth of understanding, and neither has lasting merit without it.

In the 1960s, the Zen Master Shunryu Suzuki gave a series of seminars to students in Los Altos, California. 'Each of us must make his own true way,' he said, 'and when we do, that way will express the universal way. When you understand one thing through and through, you understand everything. When you try to understand everything, you will not understand anything. The best way is to understand yourself, and then you will understand everything.'[1]

In this paradox we can discern an answer to the question begged by John Salinsky's books about books: 'Why bother?' More specifically, given all the medical textbooks, journals, guidelines and information that cascade onto our desks and screens and compete for our leisure moments, what is to be gained from time spent in a fictional universe? Will it make us better doctors? Surely it will. The novelist has the luxury of exploring and communicating a near-complete understanding of one particular microcosm, uncomplicated by real-life entanglements. To the extent that we can identify with a well-drawn fictional character, we can, as Suzuki enjoins us, understand that one 'self' through and through, and thereby hone our understanding of all the other selves we encounter professionally.

The most fundamental of all consulting skills is genuine curiosity about other people, the constant urge to wonder 'Why are they as they are?' In the words of another Zenist, Martine Batchelor, 'The most important part of the question is not the meaning of the words themselves but the question mark.'[2] We should open our minds to the life of the imagination not just for its entertainment value, but for the mindset of curiosity it engenders in us. Such books as John Salinsky describes in this and his previous volume combine powerful opportunities for our own professional growth with pleasure and recreation too. What could be better?

Roger Neighbour MA PRCGP
Former GP, Abbots Langley, Hertfordshire
President, Royal College of General Practitioners
November 2003

References

1 Suzuki S (1970) *Zen Mind, Beginner's Mind*. Weatherhill, New York.

2 Batchelor M (1999) *Principles of Zen*. Thorsons, London.

About the authors

John Salinsky is a general practitioner in Wembley, Middlesex, and course organiser at the Whittington Vocational Training Scheme for General Practice. Since 1998 he has been responsible for the 'Medicine and Literature' column in the journal *Education for Primary Care*. His first collection, *Medicine and Literature: the doctor's companion to the classics*, was published in 2002.

Gillie Bolton is senior research fellow in Medicine and the Arts at King's College, London. She has written (among other things, including 56 poems about angels) *The Therapeutic Potential of Creative Writing: writing myself, reflective practice writing and professional development* and co-edited *Writing Cures*.

Brian Glasser is a teaching fellow in the Centre for Medical Humanities at the Royal Free & University College Medical School, as well as patient information programme officer at the Royal Free Hampstead NHS Trust. He is the author of a book about Europe's most important jazz musician, entitled *In A Silent Way: a portrait of Joe Zawinul*.

Wai-Ching Leung is a doctor working in general practice and public health. He also has an interest in medical education and has written about it in the *British Medical Journal*. In the last few years he has developed a passion for literature and is now studying it for an MA degree at the Open University.

Aziz Sheikh is a part-time general practitioner and Professor of Primary Health Care Research and Development at the University of Edinburgh. His interests include epidemiology, medical ethics and exploring the interface between religion, culture and healthcare. Aziz chairs the Research and Documentation Committee of The Muslim Council of Britain.

Alistair Stead has recently retired from the School of English at the University of Leeds, where he lectured on English and American literature.

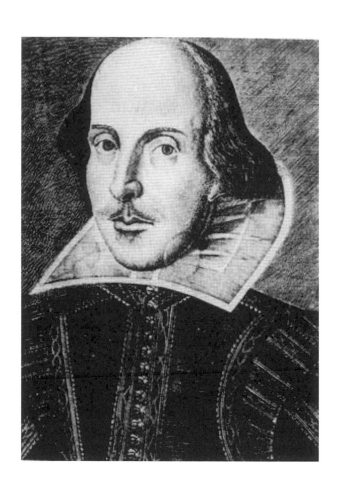

1

Introduction

It gives me great pleasure to be able to introduce a second collection of essays on some favourite literary classics, which I would like to share with you. As I said in my introduction to the first volume, I think we should read these books chiefly because they are so enjoyable. They will all provide wonderful refreshment for our spirits after a hard day in the surgery or the clinic. In addition, we may find that the classic books can give us fresh insights into the minds of the people who crowd in daily, seeking our attention. The great writers have a marvellous ability simply to describe what it is to be human: to live in a vast and sometimes unfriendly world and to share it with other human beings for whom we develop powerful and mysterious feelings.

At first sight, the characters in a classic novel may seem to live in a different universe from the patients in the consulting room. They are more heroic or more villainous; they are preoccupied with philosophical questions or caught up in terrifying obsessions. Their lives and loves and intrigues seem much more interesting and exciting than those of people in 'real life'. But if we look carefully, we find that our patients are not so different. They too have love affairs and suffer from overwhelming yearnings, desires and jealousies. They are prone to introspection and wondering why on earth a terrible blow has happened to them. They have ambitions and compulsions; they want to get rich or avenge injustice; they have their dreams and their nightmare visions. If I am getting bored or restless in a consultation, I sometimes try to detach myself and listen to my patient in a slightly different way, as if I were reading about him in a novel. Of course, it doesn't always make a difference, but when it does, it can make my sinking heart revive and beat in sympathy with that of a fellow human being. So it is my hope, and that of my fellow contributors, that you will not only enjoy reading our recommendations in your precious spare time but be able to use the experience to enhance your understanding of your patients.

Let me now tell you about the books we have chosen for this second volume. You will notice that we have introduced works by new authors (such as Joseph Conrad, Herman Melville, DH Lawrence and Virginia Woolf) and also revisited some of our old friends from the original *Medicine and Literature* to see what else they have written. William Shakespeare, Jane Austen, Leo Tolstoy and Franz Kafka make welcome reappearances, and the Brontë sisters are represented by Charlotte instead of Emily.

This time there are shorter works, which may be welcome news for those who get nervous when presented with a massive tome. However, in this collection, brevity does not mean insignificance: the short stories and novels discussed here are some of the greatest works of literature the world will ever see. We have not just one but three stories by Kafka. As well as *The Metamorphosis* (the one about the man who becomes a beetle), I will be telling you about two less well-known but equally unforgettable stories written near the end of Kafka's life. Tolstoy's *The Death of Ivan Ilyich* is a good deal shorter than *Anna Karenina*, but its impact is stunning. Conrad's *Heart of Darkness* is another compressed masterpiece, which has influenced many subsequent writers (and film makers) but remains unequalled. I would also say, in defence of great short books, that if you finish one before your journey ends, you can not do better than to start again at the beginning. You will be rewarded by fresh insights and unexpected revelations, even if you thought you had read every word.

Although the average length of the books in this volume is shorter than in the first, you will notice that many of the chapters are longer. Why should this be, I wondered. I have been writing about the classics for a few years now and during that time my approach has undergone a change. I seem to go more deeply into the books and stay there longer. I spend more time relishing the details and working out what is going on. In my presentations to my readers, I find I can no longer skim over parts of the plot that don't seem to matter. Everything now seems more likely to be there for a purpose. And there is another reason for my longer chapters. In the first volume, I wanted to share with you the books that were old favourites. This volume also contains faithful companions from the bedside table, but I have added some books by writers whom I have always respected but found difficult. I thought it was time to find out whether my increased age and exposure to life had made me more receptive. Conrad is a good example of a writer whose style I always found hard going. Perhaps that's why I chose his shortest novel to begin with. I didn't think 100 pages would detain me long, but I was wrong. I spent a long time in the jungle with the old sea captain going up that terrible river, and I was a changed person when I came out. I had seen into the depths of the abyss. I had also learned how to read very slowly. I think that was the key.

Another great writer whose books I was never able to finish in my teens is DH Lawrence. I loved the musicality of his language but was defeated by the apparent waywardness of his characters and the strangeness of his ideas. I decided to tackle *Women in Love,* which the professionals agree is his greatest and most typically Lawrentian book. *Sons and Lovers* would have been much easier but I wanted to go for the big challenge on your behalf. So I immersed myself in Lawrence's world. I learned about his life, I read his letters and what his friends and enemies have had to say about him over the years. I read some of his other books. And I really got to know those women in love (and their men). When I emerged I had added the book to my list of all time favourites. I felt almost as if I had spent time with Lawrence in person. We had been for long country walks, talked earnestly, warmed to each other, got drunk in pubs, disagreed violently, tried to understand each other and ended up as firm friends (although my other friends think he's a bit weird). I would like you to read Lawrence too, especially if you never have. I don't want you to go through as big a struggle as I did, and I hope that my personal discoveries about *Women in Love* will make the journey much easier for you than it was for me.

In complete contrast, I have also included Evelyn Waugh's *Decline and Fall*, a book that delighted me with its ruthless wit when I was an undergraduate. But when I reread it more recently,

I found there were some chapters that made me feel morally queasy. Does this mean I was wrong to enjoy it? I want you to read it too and help me to make a judgement.

So much for the literature, what about the medicine? You will by now be well aware that we do not restrict ourselves to books about doctors and patients, because all accounts of human lives will resonate with the lives of those who pass in and out of our consulting rooms. Nevertheless, doctors must and will make their appearance on the literary stage and we can't fail to be fascinated by the problems they create for themselves. Would I have behaved like that, we wonder, when a fictional doctor does something shameful and embarrassing? Surely not. Well perhaps, but only on a really bad day .... Our most spectacular fictional doctors are Victor Frankenstein and Henry Jekyll. Both of these larger-than-life colleagues will be sure to evoke your compassion even if you decide not to follow their research interests. Why is it, I wonder, that writers tend to choose a medical man when they want to portray a hero who recklessly meddles with nature and brings about catastrophe? Perhaps it is because our patients regard us with a certain ambivalence: look at the public unease over the genetic manipulation of human embryos. Some of us may combine scientific ingenuity with demonic powers. Does your kindly family doctor have a mad gleam in his eye? What is he cooking up in his home laboratory?

Disturbing in a different way is Ivan Turgenev's formidable Doctor Eugene Bazarov from *Fathers and Sons*. Strictly speaking, Bazarov is not yet fully qualified, but he is already a ruthless advocate of evidence-based medicine. And he shocks the older generation with his contemptuous dismissal of their cherished values. All the same, he is a conscientious doctor and he can be kind and generous; I think you will find that you have a soft spot for him too.

The doctor as a minor character pops up all over the place, giving us the pleasure of comparing our consultation style with his. In Jane Austen's *Emma* we shall hear about the devoted local GP, Mr Perry, whose patience with the heartsinking Mr Woodhouse will evoke your grudging admiration. Some of our other patients are not so lucky: poor Ivan Ilyich gets very indifferent palliative care from both GP and oncologist, and Virginia Woolf's Septimus Warren Smith receives deplorable treatment from the eminent psychiatrist Sir William Bradshaw. Look out for cameo doctor appearances in *Jane Eyre, Moby-Dick* and *Heart of Darkness*. Finally, we must not forget Dr Aziz in *A Passage to India*. Although we never see him at work (I'm sure he is very patient-centred) we shall be totally involved in his struggles with his own emotions and with the British Raj.

In my encounters with some of the characters described within, I have been unable to resist the temptation to play the doctor myself. You may think this is out of order, since I am not licensed to practise in their world, and most of the characters have not even declared themselves as patients. Despite these objections (which I fully accept), I have offered diagnostic speculations about Jaques (*As You Like It*), Mr Kurtz (*Heart of Darkness*), Gerald Crich (*Women in Love*) and the unnamed subterranean creature in Kafka's story *The Burrow*.

Many other deeply disturbed characters are also to be found in our chosen books. Whether they would agree to a psychiatric referral or even a few sessions with the practice counsellor I could not say. But, extreme as these people are, I feel sure that we all have patients in our surgeries and clinics who resemble them closely. Of course, they will not be consulting us about their mental state; they will be more concerned with the behaviour of their spouses, their need for our signature on a dubious document or the rebellious state of their inner organs.

Look out for Captain Ahab, who is preoccupied with a long-standing feud which he seems determined to pursue to the death. Keep a spare appointment for little Jane Eyre, whose anxiety over her reckless older boyfriend will have produced all sorts of psychosomatic symptoms. What about that poor Mr Samsa, whose life has never been the same since he woke up one morning unable to use his legs properly or to speak? Here's a Russian man worried about the dangerous friend his son has taken up with at the university. Even the strange people from *One Hundred Years of Solitude*, with their morbid obsessions, bizarre behaviour and inability to communicate, will manage to find their way through the Colombian jungle to the surgery in the clearing.

The stories and novels cover a generous time span, and this time I have placed them in chronological order. I hope you approve. The romantics of the nineteenth century are well represented, closely followed by the modernists of the early twentieth. Love, death and family relationships preoccupy many of our characters; others are caught up in the single-minded pursuit of an idea, an ambition or the thirst for revenge. The problems and moral ambiguities of Empire are discussed in *Heart of Darkness* and *A Passage to India*. The shadow of the Great War looms over *Women in Love* and *Mrs Dalloway*.

As in the previous volume, I am delighted to welcome the contributions of my fellow enthusiasts for medicine and literature. Wai-Ching Leung introduces us to Virginia Woolf's *Mrs Dalloway* and her tragic alter ego Septimus Smith. Gillie Bolton writes about Mary Shelley's *Frankenstein*, whose unhappy monster is more human than you might think. And Brian Glasser describes the 'strange case' of RL Stevenson's *Dr Jekyll and Mr Hyde* and their translation from the page to the screen. Aziz Sheikh supplies a thoughtful postscript from a different perspective to my essay on *A Passage to India*. Once again, I would like to thank Alistair Stead for his careful reading of the manuscripts and his valuable advice on everything from punctuation to interpretation. Alistair has also contributed his own postscripts to the chapters on Kafka and Tolstoy.

We begin with Shakespeare: another piece inspired by a visit with my GP registrars to the Open Air Theatre in Regent's Park, London, on a summer's evening. The stage is set so I shall not detain you any further, but, borrowing a phrase from Rosalind, I charge you to like as much of the play (and the rest of the book) as please you.

Happy reading.

2

As You Like It

by William Shakespeare (1599)

If you read the first volume of *Medicine and Literature*, you may remember that I was inspired to write about a Shakespeare comedy by a visit to the Open Air Theatre in Regent's Park, London, with my course organiser colleague Caroline Dickinson, and our little band of GP registrars. On that occasion the play was *A Midsummer Night's Dream*, and we all enjoyed it so much that 'Shakespeare in the Park' became a regular summer event. Last year we went to see *As You Like It*, and we liked it very much in spite of the chilly July weather and a brisk downpour in the first five minutes.

I wrote a synopsis for the registrars to read beforehand and it forms the basis of this account. With *A Midsummer Night's Dream* I felt obliged to pick out a few medical themes in the play; but now that we all believe in the importance of medical humanities there can no longer be any doubt that Shakespeare should be given an honoured place in the curriculum. So imagine yourselves sitting (warmly wrapped up please) in the park on an English summer's evening, full of eager anticipation. The play is about to begin.

The action is set partly in a ducal court and mainly in the idyllic landscape of the Forest of Arden. The play's themes include whether it's more fun to live in the town or the country and whether it's better to be a romantic or a cynic. But mainly it's about love.

Trouble at court: brothers behaving badly

The opening scenes of the play are used to get us up to speed with what Hollywood calls 'the back story', or what has been happening before the play begins. Shakespeare does this in a fairly obvious way by getting the characters to ask each other: 'What's the news at the new court?' The fact is that he doesn't want to waste too much effort on the machinery of the plot because his main aim is to get the characters away from court and into the Forest of Arden, where they can get in touch with their feelings.

The play starts in Duke Frederick's orchard, where we find our young hero, Orlando, complaining to his faithful old servant Adam about the shabby way his elder brother, Oliver, has treated him since their father's death. It seems that Oliver has denied him a proper education and brought him up as a peasant instead of a gentleman. Adam listens patiently, like the good old retainer he is. A little later in the scene we learn, from a conversation between Oliver and Charles, the court wrestler, that the old Duke (Senior) has been deposed by his younger brother Frederick and banished to the country. Several sympathetic lords have gone with him, but his daughter, Rosalind, has been allowed to stay at court because of her close friendship with her cousin Celia, the bad Duke's daughter. Charles the wrestler tells Oliver that his little brother is planning to get into the ring with him at tomorrow's tournament. Charles doesn't think this is wise and is worried that he might kill or maim Orlando. But wicked old Oliver says by all means kill him: 'I would as lief you did break his neck as his finger'.

Two girls watch a wrestling match

In scene two, we meet the two cousins, Rosalind and Celia. Rosalind is a little subdued because her father, the old Duke, has just been banished. They have an encounter with Touchstone, the court jester, who engages them in some very obscure Shakespearian clown banter about pancakes and mustard. It's not actually very funny but I promise you his act improves after he has had a chance to warm up.

Then they get ready for the wrestling. They hear that the fearsome Charles has already crushed the ribs of three young brothers, and when Orlando appears the girls try to persuade him not to fight. Naturally, Orlando insists on going on with the bout and we actually get to watch. I don't know what sort of wrestling they did at the Globe in Shakespeare's time, but modern producers tend to go for American-style dirty wrestling of the kind that you may come across as you flick idly through the more disreputable cable or satellite TV channels. There are usually lots of drop kicks, forearm jabs and Boston crabs. I can't imagine where I learned all these terms. The fight is very realistic and quite exciting and, against all the odds, it is Orlando who wins. The girls are thrilled, and Rosalind gives him her chain to wear around his neck. She is very taken with him, and in our production their eyes meet meaningfully for several tingling seconds. Rosalind really would like to hang around and chat to him a bit longer, but Celia tugs her away. Orlando is furious with himself for becoming stupefied and forgetting all his usual chat-up lines.

When the two girls are alone, Rosalind goes very quiet and Celia realises that she has fallen in love. She tries a few puns to get her to lighten up a bit ('come, come, wrestle with thy affections') but Rosalind is seriously smitten. Just then the bad Duke (Celia's father) appears and tells Rosalind that she is banished too and should pack her bags at once. Celia says that she and Rosalind are inseparable, and if Rosalind has to go, Celia will jolly well go with her. Worsted by the two teenagers, the Duke stalks off angrily while our heroines resolve to join Rosalind's father and his merry men in the Forest of Arden. Rosalind decides that, for their greater protection, she will dress up as a boy and call herself 'Ganymede'. 'Now go we in consent,' says Celia, 'to liberty and not to banishment.'

Into the forest

Now we have reached Act 2 and the scene changes to the magical Forest of Arden. You can really feel the stress dissolving away as we leave the sordid intrigues and vicious plots of the court behind us. The season is probably winter but spring is just around the corner – and so is love. The good old banished Duke (Rosalind's father) is telling his friends how much better life will be in the woods and fields. It's true that the winter wind can bite 'as the icy fang' when you are in the great outdoors, but no matter. We shall find, he says, 'tongues in trees, books in the running brooks, sermons in stones, and good in everything'. One of the nice things about watching a Shakespeare play is that you keep hearing and happily recognising wonderful quotations. There will be lots more in this play and I will be glad to signpost a few of them.

Meanwhile, back at the Court, the wicked Duke Frederick orders a search party to bring back the runaway girls and also to round up Orlando, who, he is led to believe, has gone to join them. The faithful servant Adam warns Orlando to get out of town quick and offers to come with him. Orlando wonders what they will do for money. Old Adam rather recklessly offers the young master the sum of 500 crowns, which must represent his entire pension fund. And so, more than adequately resourced, our young man and his old companion set off to join the other fugitives in the country.

Cutting swiftly back to the forest, we come upon Rosalind and Celia, accompanied by Touchstone, the clown. Rosalind is now disguised as a boy and we are meant to accept the convention that not even her father or her lover can recognise her. I will remind you that, at the Globe Theatre, the women's parts were all played by boys, which may account for the frequency of cross-dressing by Shakespearian heroines. However, our Rosalind's trousers, leather braces and short haircut will only enhance her feminine appeal in the best pantomime principal boy tradition. All the men in the audience will be in love with her and, I dare say, some of the women too. And the gay men will be in love with *him*, if you see what I mean.

Act 3: town versus country

In the next few scenes we have more opportunities to watch the court folk reacting to life in the country. Now we have a little musical interlude ('Under the greenwood tree, Who loves to lie with me') provided by a singer called Amiens, who is part of the Duke's travelling entourage. Listening to the song is the gloomy courtier, Jaques (pronounced Jay-queese). He cajoles Amiens to sing some more. The singer warns him: 'It will make you melancholy, Monsieur Jaques.' But Jaques replies, 'I can suck melancholy out of a song, as a weasel sucks eggs. More, I prithee, more.'

Later, when the Duke and the courtiers wander in, Jaques tells them about his meeting in the forest with Touchstone, and says he wouldn't mind being a licensed fool himself so that he could make fun of people and expose their sins and follies with impunity. Then he could 'cleanse the foul body of th'infected world'. The Duke observes that his friend was something of a hell raiser himself in his younger days and can scarcely claim to be pure. Jaques is not lost for a reply, but I think the thrust goes home. What are we to make of Jaques? He seems to be one of those very clever and rather unnerving people who stand around at parties making satirical remarks but never getting involved. He always has something smart to say about human weakness and he appears to be very cynical and sneering. But underneath the mask he is quite vulnerable. He is always called 'melancholy', and I think he is quite depressed. His saving grace is that he still finds the world interesting.

Now who is this staggering dramatically into the forest clearing to interrupt the Duke's picnic? It is Orlando, who is tired, hungry and desperate. At first he demands food with menaces; but the Duke assures him that he is welcome to join them and he calms down. Orlando asks permission to go and get Adam, whom he has left, exhausted, a little further back. The truth is that while Adam is very game, he is over 80, for goodness sake, and is really a bit too decrepit to be taken on strenuous hikes through the forest.

The seven ages of man: a jaundiced view?

At this point Jaques comes out with his famous 'Seven Ages of Man' speech, which many of us had to learn at school and can still recite fragments of. I am sure you remember that it starts with 'the infant mewling and puking in the nurse's arms' and proceeds via the reluctant schoolboy, the sighing lover, the swearing soldier, the fat pompous justice and 'the lean and slippered pantaloon' to the final late geriatric stage: 'sans eyes, sans teeth, sans taste, sans everything'. In the production we saw, this last line is delivered with a meaning look at old Adam, who is lying on the ground, looking more dead than alive. However, he does recover, and is able to tuck into some much-needed breakfast. So is Jaques' depressing version of the human life story to be taken seriously? In each of the seven ages, human beings are seen as being miserable or ruthlessly self-serving or both. As a later cynic put it: 'Life is shit and then you die.'

But it doesn't have to be like that, does it? I mean, it's true you die in the end, but you can have a lot of fun along the way and even feel you have achieved a thing or two before it's time to meet your maker, if indeed that is what happens. I think we doctors all see someone like Jaques in the surgery now and then and find him very entertaining. But when he goes on his lonely way again we feel a tinge of sadness. Perhaps he needs some cognitive behavioural therapy.

Love poems on the trees

Now, I am happy to say, the mood changes and the romantic comedy really gets going. Who is this hanging love poems on all the trees and incising them on their trunks? It is young Orlando, who is now looking forward to a different and more delightful kind of wrestling. But before we get Rosalind's response, Shakespeare deftly inserts the cynical view with a conversation between Touchstone and Corin, an old shepherd. Corin praises the innocence of country life, but Touchstone (whose wit is warming up in the sun) points out that a shepherd is little better than a brothel-keeper who earns his living by procuring young she-lambs for dirty old rams.

Now enter Rosalind (in her boy's clothes) and Celia to find the trees covered with rather bad verses in praise of Rosalind:

From the east to western Ind,
No jewel is like Rosalind.

And Touchstone mockingly offers:

If a hart do lack a hind,
Let him seek out Rosalind.

Celia reads out a long verse and Rosalind pretends to be embarrassed (although she is really quite excited). She demands to know who the writer is, and Celia, after some teasing, reveals that he is Orlando. Rosalind is impatient and full of questions: 'What said he? How looked he? Wherein went he? What makes he here? Did he ask for me? Where remains he? How parted he with thee? And when shalt thou see him again? Answer me in one word.'

When Orlando himself appears, Rosalind decides to keep her male identity for the time being ('I will speak to him like a saucy lackey') and test the strength of Orlando's love; always a prudent thing for a girl to do. She teases the poor boy with some amazing wordplay (or is it foreplay?). She dazzles him with a brilliant speech about the way time moves at different speeds for different people: 'I'll tell you who Time ambles withal, who Time trots withal, who Time gallops withal, and who he stands still withal.'

She tells him that he can't really be in love because he doesn't look the part. Everyone knows that a young man in love has:

a lean cheek, which you have not; a blue eye and sunken, which you
have not; an unquestionable spirit, which you have not; a beard neg-
lected, which you have not .... Then your hose should be ungartered,
your bonnet unbanded, your sleeve unbuttoned, your shoe untied,
and everything about you demonstrating a careless desolation. But you
are no such man: you are rather point-device in your accoutrements, as
loving yourself, than seeming the lover of any other.

Girls, whenever you encounter a young fellow who is really sharply dressed, without a hair out of place, you should confuse him by telling him that he is 'point-device in his accoutrements'.

Bending the gender

Orlando protests that he really is in love with Rosalind (whom, of course, he fails to recognise in her trousers). The strange youth offers to cure him of love by a special form of therapy. He will have to play a game in which 'Ganymede' pretends to be Rosalind and gives Orlando a really hard time by constantly changing 'her' moods: 'now like him, now loathe him; then entertain him, then forswear him, now weep for him, then spit at him'. Orlando says he doesn't want to be cured, but he accepts the offer 'with all my heart, good youth'. 'Nay,' says his mentor, 'you must call me Rosalind.'

Orlando goes along with the charade, ensuring that the fun continues. But is he really fooled? He must 'know' at some unconscious level that Ganymede is really Rosalind. Let me confuse you further by reminding you that Rosalind/Ganymede was played by a boy actor until the Restoration, when women actors were allowed on the stage for the first time. They seized joyfully on the part of Rosalind and naturally have been unwilling to give it up ever since, although there have recently been some all-male productions of As You Like It. Being disguised as a boy liberates Rosalind and enables her to take the leading role in the relationship. Orlando was in love with her when she was a conventional young woman, but he must be even more entranced with this witty, pretty, sparkling, energetic boy-girl with a heart – just as we all are.

So is he in love with a boy or a girl? And does she appeal to a gay, boy-loving part of his nature? Or is her boyishness essentially feminine, whatever that means? And what difference does it make if, as in Shakespeare's time, Rosalind is 'really' a boy? I shall return to the gender question before we finish, but meanwhile, don't bother your pretty heads about it – just enjoy the show.

More lovers and their problems

Next we have an interlude for another pair of lovers. Touchstone, the jester, has found himself a simple country wench called

Audrey, whom he is determined to marry, quite undeterred by the major differences in their interests and background. I am afraid he is rather coarse and lacking in spirituality. Audrey seems not to mind.

We then take a look at a third, and rather stormy, relationship, that of Silvius, the young shepherd, and Phebe, a shepherdess, who does not (yet) return his affections. Rosalind (as Ganymede) gives Phebe a good telling off for being too proud to accept an offer from such a fine young fellow as Silvius. She tells Phebe bluntly that a girl in her position is not likely to find anyone better in a rural community. 'Down on your knees,' she admonishes, 'and thank heaven, fasting, for a good man's love.' Is Rosalind really giving herself the same advice? At any rate, the unexpected result is that poor little Phebe immediately gets a crush on Ganymede/Rosalind: 'I had rather hear you chide than this man woo.' 'I pray you do not fall in love with me,' retorts Rosalind, 'for I am falser than vows made in wine. Besides I like you not.' Well, that's plain enough. But, of course, the besotted Phebe takes no notice. True, Ganymede has been rather rough with her, but he is *very* good looking. She tells poor Silvius (now reduced to the role of confidant) that some girls might have fallen in love with such a devastatingly rude youth but not her: she is going to write Ganymede a scathing letter (which Silvius is to deliver).

Act 4: a lesson in love

Orlando turns up a little late for his first appointment with the love therapist, whom he still fails to recognise as his Rosalind. After warning him not to be late again, she relents and gets him to practise his love talk: 'Come woo me, woo me: for now I am in a holiday humour and like enough to consent. What would you say to me now, an I were your very, very Rosalind?' Orlando says, 'I would kiss before I spoke', which is a good answer, and the lesson goes really well. 'Rosalind' proposes a mock marriage, with Celia officiating as priest. Rosalind warns him that she will be a very jealous and often annoying wife. Orlando is not a bit discouraged. Then he says he must be excused for two hours while he has dinner with the Duke. Rosalind pretends to be disillusioned with him and makes him promise not to be late back. After he has gone, Celia reproves Rosalind for bringing the female sex into disrepute by her antics. In a famous, heart-stopping revelation of her true feelings, Rosalind comes back with: 'O coz, coz, my pretty little coz, that thou didst know how many fathoms deep I am in love!'

After another interlude for a song, events move on quickly. Silvius presents Rosalind with Phebe's 'chiding' letter – which is really a declaration of love. Rosalind tells Silvius to make a more determined pitch for Phebe himself and not be 'a tame snake'. Now in comes Orlando's wicked elder brother Oliver, with a rather improbable tale to tell. It seems that while he was asleep under an oak tree, a lioness crept up on him and would have killed him had not young Orlando leapt out to his defence and killed the animal in fierce single combat. Perhaps the Forest of Arden is a more dangerous place than we thought. Orlando was wounded by the lioness's claws and Oliver had to staunch the flow of blood. He shows them 'the bloody napkin' as proof and tells the two girls that Orlando has asked him to show it to 'the shepherd youth That he in sport doth call his "Rosalind" '. The sight of her beloved's blood makes Rosalind faint, but when she recovers she quickly tells Oliver that this was merely a 'counterfeit'. Nobody is fooled. Touched by his brother's heroism, bad Oliver now becomes good Oliver and is free to fall in love with Celia, who has been left single for long enough.

Act 5: all to be married tomorrow

In the first scene of the final act, we see the brothers Orlando and Oliver happily reconciled after their adventure with the lioness. Oliver is going to marry Celia the following day, and Orlando is getting impatient for some satisfaction of his own desire. 'I can live no longer by thinking,' he says, miserably. But 'Ganymede' (alias Rosalind) tells him she 'can do strange things' and he too will be married tomorrow. Silvius now enters with Phebe, who is still mooning over Ganymede and breaking her young shepherd's heart. Silvius tells us, with simple, moving eloquence 'what love is':

Silvius:	*It is to be all made of sighs and tears;*
	And so am I for Phebe.
Phebe:	*And I for Ganymede.*
Orlando:	*And I for Rosalind.*
Rosalind:	*And I for no woman.*

Silvius loves Phebe, Phebe loves Rosalind (whom she thinks is a boy) and Rosalind cunningly says she is in love 'with no woman'. The others all think it's a mess. But Rosalind is in complete control of the plot and she confidently guarantees that everyone will be appropriately paired off and married the next day. Her last word to Phebe is 'I will marry you if ever I marry woman, and I'll be married tomorrow.'

Of course, as we in the audience know, it's not really all that difficult. All Rosalind has to do is to change back into a frock and everything will become clear. But before that happens Shakespeare throws in a few more diversions for our enjoyment. Two pages sing a well-known song ('It was a lover and his lass'). Then Touchstone introduces his bride-to-be, Audrey, to Jaques and the Duke, describing her rather unkindly as 'a poor virgin, sir, an ill-favoured thing, sir, but mine own'. Touchstone follows with a final set piece of jester's wit, describing the seven phases of a quarrel and how to avoid a quarrel turning into a fight. It's full of wonderful technical terms such as 'the Reproof Valiant' and 'the Countercheck Quarrelsome'.

At last Rosalind and Celia reappear and Rosalind is again wearing a skirt (sad to say). All four couples are now appropriately united in a ceremony performed by 'a masquer' representing Hymen, the Roman god of marriage. In a final piece of plot-spinning good news, we are told that the bad Duke Frederick has now seen the error of his ways (he was 'converted' by 'an old religious man' whom he met in the forest) and is now happy to let the good Duke Senior reclaim the crown. So that's all right. We don't have to stay in the forest, we can all go back to court and live happily in comfort. Only Jaques decides that it would be more interesting to stay and chat to the born-again, formerly evil, Duke Frederick. As I told you, Shakespeare simply can't be bothered with subtle plotting in this play. But he rounds it off beautifully by clearing the stage and having Rosalind step forward to deliver a saucy epilogue. 'It is not the fashion,' she begins, 'to see the lady the epilogue ...' – but note that she is back in her trousers and braces, teasing us with those gender questions again. She speaks first to the women and then to the men:

> I charge you, O women, for the love you bear to men, to like as much of this play as please you; and I charge you, O men, for the love you bear to women – as I perceive by your simpering, none of you hates them – that between you and the women the play may please. If I were a woman, I would kiss as many of you as had beards that pleased me, complexions that liked me, and breaths that I defied not; and, I am sure, as many as have good beards, or good faces, or sweet breaths, will, for my kind offer, when I make curtsy, bid me farewell.

Finally

I do urge you to see the play, too: I am certain that it will please you, as it's difficult not to succumb to its allure. It's a lot of fun, but is it serious as well? Or was it just written to entertain the Elizabethan crowd and get the new Globe Theatre off to a brilliant start in 1599? I think it was certainly intended to be a terrific show and to satirise the fashion for sentimental, pastoral love stories. But it also leaves me reflecting that it takes someone as wise as Rosalind (whether boy or girl or a bit of both) to understand what love is all about. And I think that the unremarkable Orlando is lucky to have found someone as wise and witty and loving as Rosalind.

The text

As You Like It is available in The New Penguin Shakespeare edition, edited, with an introduction and notes, by HJ Oliver.

3

Emma

by Jane Austen (1816)

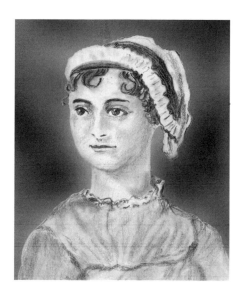

Introduction

'I am going to take a heroine whom no one but myself will much like,' said Jane Austen, writing to her sister about the fifth of her great sextet of novels. The girl in question was Emma Woodhouse and, in fact, everyone loved her, as Jane probably knew they would. Unlike shy, nervous little Fanny Price of *Mansfield Park*, Emma has bags of self-confidence. And while Fanny has an unerring moral sense and always does the right thing, this is not the case with Emma. Perhaps that's why we readers are so fond of her. (I love Fanny too, but in a different way, more protectively.)

Here, to show you how easy it is to read Jane Austen, is the first sentence of *Emma*, introducing our wayward heroine:

> *Emma Woodhouse, handsome, clever and rich, with a comfortable home and happy disposition, seemed to unite some of the best blessings of existence; and had lived nearly twenty-one years in the world with very little to distress or vex her.*

Reading on, we learn that Emma lives with her elderly father in a peaceful village called Highbury, in the county of Surrey (or 'Surry' as Jane calls it). Highbury is 16 miles from London and is somewhere near Dorking. Emma's mother died when she was an infant and she has been brought up since the age of 5 by a governess called Miss Taylor, who must have been an excellent mother-substitute, because Emma seems untouched by maternal deprivation.

Enter Mr Knightley

But now Miss Taylor has gone and got married to a young widower called Mr Weston (everyone is addressed quite formally in Highbury, but you will soon get used to it). Emma's father regards this marriage as quite deplorable: 'Ah! Poor Miss Taylor! 'tis a sad business.' Mr Woodhouse is a very self-centred chap, pre-occupied almost entirely with his own comfort. This is amusing at first, but some readers develop a hearty dislike for the old boy. Emma misses her mother-substitute of course, but is comforted by the fact that she and her husband are living only half a mile away. During our first evening at Hartfield (the house and grounds belonging to Emma's father) we also meet Mr Knightley, a friend of the family, who has walked over from his rather stately home a mile away. (He is always known as 'Mr Knightley', although his name is George. He has a brother called John, who is married to Emma's elder sister, Isabella. Now draw a family tree.) Mr Knightley is 'a sensible man about seven or eight-and-thirty'. So he is quite a bit older than Emma, and we soon discover that they have a rather special relationship. They are clearly fond of each other, but Mr K sees it as his duty to try and correct some of his young friend's impulsive behaviour. 'Mr Knightley was in fact one of the few people who could see faults in Emma Woodhouse, and the only one who ever told her about them.' What sort of faults, one wonders? Then we hear Emma claiming to have 'made the match' between her governess and Mr Weston. Her father says he would rather she didn't make any more matches, 'for whatever you say always comes to pass'. But Emma says matchmaking is 'the greatest amusement in the world' and tells the two men how she knew from the start that Mr Weston would marry again, and how she planned that he would marry Miss Taylor. Mr Knightley, instead of being amused, puts Emma down quite sharply: 'Why do you talk of success? Where is your merit? What are you proud of? – you made a lucky guess; and that is all that can be said.' Now you will notice that Emma is not at all daunted by this reprimand; she goes on to tease him with her plans to select a wife for Mr Elton, a young clergyman recently arrived in Highbury. So what are we to make of the Emma–Knightley relationship? Here we have a spirited young woman and an older, but attractive, man, who has decided to take charge of her education and moral development. I'm thinking Eliza Doolittle and Professor Higgins, Dr Who and his succession of young female assistants, Buffy the vampire slayer and Giles, her watcher and … I am sure you can think of lots of other examples. So is there an erotic charge sparking between these two? For the moment, my lips are sealed.

Chapter 2 relates the back story of Mr Weston's first marriage. His first wife died tragically young and their son, Frank, was brought up by her brother and his wife, the Churchills, and has taken their surname. We shall meet Frank Churchill later on and puzzle over his mysterious role in the story. The only other thing I should tell you about Chapter 2 is that it includes the first mention of Highbury's leading family doctor, Mr Perry the apothecary, who will, I fear, spend far too much of his time on clinically inappropriate house calls to Emma's hypochondriacal father.

Emma and her friend Harriet: social nuances in Highbury

Chapter 3 introduces Emma's friend and protégée, the 17-year-old Harriet Smith, who plays an important role in the first part of the story. Harriet is described as being 'the natural daughter of somebody'. The somebody is probably a gentleman, because he can afford to pay for her to be a boarder at a respectable little school. Harriet is cute and pretty, but her status is precarious. Social class is terribly important in the little world of Highbury. It's not just a matter of upper, middle and lower, there are some very fine subdivisions and everyone needs to be placed very precisely at their proper level, especially where marriage is concerned. You can make a good marriage by finding someone a little higher in the hierarchy; but aim too high or sink too low and Society will not forgive you. Birth is important, so is education, and wealth is very helpful. Good manners go with status, but can even improve it to some extent. No one suggests that love might conquer all or that it would be a good thing to rebel against class-consciousness. How should we modern readers regard Highbury's social attitudes? Like anthropologists, I suggest: we need to immerse ourselves in the culture to understand the people we are living with, at least until it's time to write up the research.

So how does Harriet fit into the social scheme? Rather insecurely, I'm afraid. But she's a pleasant enough girl, eager to please, and Emma has decided to take her in hand with the idea of improving her. Harriet is delighted to be noticed by Emma, because the Woodhouses are pretty top-notch society in Highbury. Only Mr Knightley has a slightly higher rating.

Anyway, class distinctions apart, the girls enjoy spending time together. In Chapter 4 Harriet tells Emma about her friendship with a family of local farmers called the Martins, and especially with young Robert Martin, who has clearly taken a fancy to her. But Emma is very discouraging. Robert Martin may be a respectable chap, but as a farmer he is little better than a peasant. 'To be sure,' says Harriet, in a mortified voice, 'he is not so genteel as a real gentleman.' Emma kindly points out that Harriet has had the chance to observe a few 'real' gentlemen during her visits to Hartfield. There is, for example, Mr Elton, the unattached young clergyman, a very good specimen of male gentility, whose manners are improving all the time. Emma is rather like an estate agent steering a client towards a well-maintained, not-too-expensive property in an up-and-coming neighbourhood. Her intentions are good and she genuinely wishes Harriet well – but she can't resist meddling.

In the next chapter, we find Mr Knightley talking to Mrs Weston (Emma's former governess and mother-substitute) and taking a dim view of the friendship between Emma and Harriet. 'I think they will neither of them do the other any good.' Mrs Weston thinks that educating Harriet might encourage Emma to read more herself. To which Emma's self-appointed tutor replies, 'Emma has been meaning to read more ever since she was twelve years old. I have seen a great many lists ... of books that she meant to read regularly through – and very good lists they were – very well chosen .... But I have done with expecting any course of steady reading from Emma.' Oh dear. Sounds like a GP trainer lamenting the lack of application of a registrar. But a little later on, he is confiding in Mrs Weston: 'I should like to see Emma in love and in some doubt of a return; it would do her good. But there is nobody hereabouts to attach her. And she goes so seldom from home.' Hmm. Interesting. Mrs Weston gives her opinion that it's too soon for Emma to be thinking of marriage (with her father to look after and all) and Mr Knightley deftly changes the subject: 'What does Weston think of the weather; shall we have rain?' A brilliant ending to a superb Austen chapter.

Harriet has her portrait painted

Meanwhile, Emma pursues her scheme of uniting Harriet with Mr Elton. This rather wet young man now makes his appearance and compliments Emma on her work in 'improving' Harriet. Emma takes this as a definite hint of romantic interest in her pupil and offers to draw a portrait of Harriet. Mr Elton thinks this is a wonderful idea, but the truth is that he is attracted to the artist rather than the sitter. Although this is obvious to us, Emma, in her single-minded concentration on the Harriet campaign, fails to see it. We get the impression that our heroine is not especially gifted in the art department. Her beginnings are better than her finished work. The same is true of her music it seems. Emma, if only you would practise regularly. (Oh dear, I sound just like Mr Knightley.)

As soon as the portrait is finished, Mr Elton gallops off with it to London to have it framed. 'What a precious deposit!' he says as he receives it. He is a silly little man. And even Emma thinks: 'This man is almost too gallant to be in love.'

A very good letter

The next chapter (Chapter 7) concerns Robert Martin's letter. Yes, the young farmer, unaware of Emma's view of his lack of social position, has sent Harriet a written proposal of marriage. To Emma's surprise it is quite well written. She acknowledges that it is a good letter: 'so good a letter, Harriet, that everything considered, I think one of his sisters must have helped him'. What shall she do? asks Harriet anxiously. Emma replies: 'You must answer it of course – and speedily.' 'Yes. But what shall I say? Dear Miss Woodhouse, do advise me.' 'I shall not give you any advice, Harriet. I will have nothing to do with it. This is a point which you must settle with your own feelings.' But this half-hearted attempt at non-directive counselling easily breaks down and poor Harriet is soon writing a polite refusal under Emma's supervision. Robert Martin is a very decent fellow and he really loves Harriet, while to Emma she is only a plaything. When Harriet shows signs of regretting the decision to turn him down, Emma reinforces it by telling Harriet that had she agreed to marry the farmer it would have been the end of their friendship because there is no way that someone of Miss Woodhouse's stand-ing could associate with a farmer's wife. It's all very entertaining, but I can't help feeling sorry for Harriet (she's only 17) and quite cross with Emma.

Emma the matchmaker

When he learns about the letter and Emma's part in the reply, Mr Knightley is cross with her too. He points out that Harriet is really very vulnerable socially, with no family and no money. And, he adds, if Emma is plotting to make a match between Harriet and Mr Elton she will soon discover that while he is 'a very good sort of man and a respectable vicar', he is 'not at all likely to make an imprudent match'. Mr Elton, says he, will be looking for a girl who has twenty thousand pounds to her name. And he strides off angrily. Emma is a little disconcerted, but sticks to her plan and continues her efforts to bring 'the lovers' together. In sharing Emma's thoughts with us, Jane Austen uses Emma's language, but in the third person so that she can also let us know that she thinks Emma is deluding herself. This technique of free indirect speech, which enters the character's mind but allows the author to retain control of the narrative, was one of Jane Austen's brilliant literary innovations.

Next we have a visit from Emma's sister, Isabella, with her husband, Mr John Knightley (who is Mr George Knightley's brother), and their five children. Emma and her Mr Knightley make up and become friends again (although they continue arguing about who was right). Then, we have an exciting medical interlude: old Mr Woodhouse and his elder daughter, Isabella, have a family dispute about whose doctor gives the best advice. Isabella and her family have just had a holiday in South End (as they call it), where the sea bathing has done wonders for little Bella's sore throat. Either that or the embrocation prescribed by their doctor in London, Mr Wingfield. Her father is very dubious about this Wingfield. His doctor, Mr Perry, says the seaside is very unlikely to be good for your health, but if you must go it should be to Cromer, where the air is much better than at South End.

Christmas Eve at the Westons

The next major event is a Christmas Eve get-together at the Westons, half a mile away. The weather is getting colder and there is talk of snow. Harriet is unable to go because she has a sore throat. Emma thinks that Mr Elton will cry off as well, but he seems determined not to miss the party. Mr Weston talks about his son, Frank Churchill, who is shortly to pay his father and stepmother a visit. In spite of her 'resolution of never marrying', Emma might just possibly consider young Frank, who seems 'the very person to suit her in age, character and condition'. Emma has never met him but she has heard a lot about him. As she listens to the news about Frank she is aware of Mr Elton, who sits next to her at dinner, paying her a lot of attention. And it gets worse. On the way home she has to share a carriage with him. Mr Elton makes the most of his opportunity and passionately declares his love for Emma. Emma is appalled. Not only is this horrible man indifferent to Harriet, but he thinks that she, Emma, has been encouraging him! She disillusions him quickly. It's very uncomfortable being so close to him in the carriage, but 'their straightforward emotions left no room for the little zigzags of embarrassment'. Back in the safety of Hartfield she is able to review recent events and consider her mistakes. After some re-flection, she cheers up and decides things are not too bad. Harriet and Mr Elton will recover from their disappointments and the snow which is now covering the ground will prevent her from having to meet either of them for the next few days.

Harriet sheds a few tears and is comforted by Emma. Mr Elton pushes off to Bath and disappears from our story for a while. Frank Churchill (Mr Weston's son) cancels his visit to Highbury because his uncle and aunt 'cannot spare him'. Mr Knightley is disgusted, and tells Emma that he is 'a very weak young man' who is just making excuses so that he doesn't have to interrupt his pleasurable pursuits to visit his newly married father. Emma, who still sees the missing Frank as a possible husband, once again disagrees with her mentor.

A visit to the Bates's

Now we are on our way, with Emma and Harriet, to pay a call on an old lady called Mrs Bates, and her unmarried daughter, Miss Bates. The Bates ladies like to be visited and everyone agrees they are delightful, except Emma, who thinks of them as 'tiresome women'. The chief problem is that Miss Bates, the daughter, never stops talking and it's mainly nonsense. And she will go on about her niece, Jane Fairfax, who is pretty and accomplished and might be some sort of threat to Emma's position as Princess of Highbury if she ever put in an appearance.

It's true that Miss Bates does rattle on for several pages once she gets going, but in Jane Austen's hands her free association is very entertaining. She tells Emma all about her niece's latest letter, in which Jane reports that she has been ill, but not too seriously. Emma surmises that Jane's illness is the result of a disappointment in love and is quite intrigued. Furthermore, Jane is about to pay a visit, and so, in the next chapter, we get filled in on the past history of this mysterious young woman.

Who is this Jane Fairfax?

So we learn that Jane is an orphan: her father was an officer, who was killed in action, and her mother (Miss Bates's younger sister) died when Jane was three. A soldier friend of her father's, Colonel Campbell, has kindly taken her into his family and provided her with a good education. But he can't afford to settle any money on her and the expectation is that she will have to support herself by becoming a governess – a rather gloomy outlook because, in English literature, being a governess is regarded as a kind of living death. We will not dwell on the details of the romantic disappointment – which may only be gossip – but eavesdrop on Emma's thoughts again. Why, she wonders, does she dislike Jane so much? She hasn't even seen her for two years. Mr Knightley once told her the reason was because she saw in Jane 'the really accomplished young woman, which she wanted to be thought herself'.

Really, Mr Knightley can be insufferable with his clever insights. Does he always have to be right? Sometimes I wonder why Emma puts up with him. When Jane reappears she is indeed very good-looking and elegant. But bearing in mind her recent disappointment and the sad fate that awaits her (having to be a governess), Emma determines to like Jane and be nice to her. However, Jane proves to be rather cool and unforthcoming about herself – and also about her acquaintance with that other eagerly anticipated visitor, Frank Churchill.

Frank Churchill arrives at last

Frank Churchill at last descends on Highbury and Emma is not disappointed. He's a good-looking chap and he's easy to talk to. The two young people spend some time together. Emma, inquisitive as ever, wants to know what he thinks about Jane Fairfax and is interested to find that Frank, while admitting her fine qualities, always has something slightly disparaging to say about her. Her complexion is too pale, for one thing, and he agrees with Emma that she is very reserved and 'One cannot love a reserved person.'

The Emma–Frank relationship seems to be developing really well, when suddenly, the very next day, he disappears off to London to have a haircut. That's a journey of 16 miles each way. Is this mere frivolity? Or is it an excuse for some activity he wishes to conceal? We shall see. At any rate, he's back the next day and Emma thinks none the worse of him, although Mr Knightley mutters from behind his newspaper, 'Hum! Just the silly, trifling fellow I took him for.' Could he be suffering a pang of jealousy?

The next big event is a dinner party to be hosted by Mr and Mrs Cole. They are a recently arrived couple who, despite the disadvantage of a background in trade, are rising rapidly in social position so that it is just about OK, even for Emma, to accept their invitation. Her father urges her to come back early. Mr Weston protests that this will break up the party, but Emma's father thinks that 'The sooner every party breaks up, the better.' I have a sneaking sympathy with him there. In the event, the Coles' party is a great success. Everyone is there, the food is good and there is some interesting gossip. Jane Fairfax has been presented, by an unknown benefactor, with a magnificent new piano. Mrs Cole has seen it on a visit to the Bates's. Then Mrs Weston starts telling Emma of her suspicions that Mr Knightley might be planning to marry Jane. Emma finds this both improbable and alarming. She wants Mr Knightley to stay just the way he is. And so, for the time being, do we. The two girls sing and play the piano; Emma and Frank have a couple of dances and she enjoys herself, especially when Frank confides that her dancing is much better than Jane's.

Now the young people are eager to have some more dancing. There is a good deal of discussion about the most suitable venue. Should it be the Westons' house (a little too cramped) or the large room at the Crown Inn (might be a little too cold)? Old Mr Woodhouse is terrified of anyone being exposed to cold and going down with a possibly fatal illness. Emma reminds him that Dr Perry always said that wrapping up well was an excellent protection. This worked very well when little Emma had the measles. And Dr Perry visited her four times a day for a week! (Doesn't he have any other patients? What is the man thinking of?)

In the event, the ball has to be postponed because Frank Churchill is summoned back to London, where his aunt is unwell. He bids Emma a fond farewell and she decides that he must be in love with her and she a little bit in love with him. On reflection, in his absence, she decides that he is a bit unreliable and that if their love were to be a temporary diversion she would not really mind in the least. She even considers encouraging Frank to transfer his attentions to Harriet.

Meet Mrs Elton

Emma has an early opportunity to meet the vicar's new wife and a quarter of an hour's conversation is enough to convince her that Mrs Elton is 'insufferable'. She talks too much; she is vain and vulgar. She boasts about her rich brother, Mr Suckling, and his gracious home at Maple Grove. Then she offers to do Emma a big favour by introducing her to some of her well-connected friends in Bath, and, worst of all, she refers to Mr Knightley as 'Knightley' and compliments him on being 'quite the gentleman'. I don't know if you listen to *The Archers*, but if you do, think of Linda Snell on a bad day and you will immediately hear the sound of Augusta Elton's voice (smarmy with a hint of menace). After she takes her gracious leave, Emma is seething with fury: 'A little upstart vulgar being' she calls her, and goes on at some length. Of course, for us, Mrs Elton is a very entertaining addition to the cast and we enjoy seeing Emma spitting with rage. Mrs Elton's next offence is to take a meddlesome interest in Jane Fairfax. She wants to invite her to dinner and introduce her to friends, which is not so bad, but she also has plans to find poor Jane a post as a governess. ('My acquaintance is so very extensive that I have little doubt of hearing of something to suit her shortly.')

Jane's trip to the post office

In view of future developments, I must draw your attention now to a little episode in which Jane Fairfax slips down to the post office on a very rainy morning. Kindly, health-conscious Mr Woodhouse is very concerned about the consequences of her getting wet: 'Young ladies should take care of themselves – young ladies are delicate plants. They should take care of their health and their complexion. My dear, did you change your stockings?' Mrs Elton butts in with her customary interference and says that in future she will arrange for Jane's letter to be brought to her. But who is the correspondent whose letters Jane is so anxious to receive? Have you guessed yet? There are plenty of clues scattered about and this is sometimes referred to as the 'detective story' in *Emma*.

Mrs Elton continues to go on at Jane about the need to get fixed up with a job as soon as possible. Jane, who is in no hurry, compares the trade in governesses with the slave trade, but Mrs Elton assures her she will find her a superior situation where she can 'mix in the family as much as you choose'. We are treated to many more examples of Mrs Elton's cringe-making conversation. I particularly like the way she disgusts Emma by referring to her father as 'this dear old beau of mine … I wish you had heard his gallant speeches at dinner. Oh I assure you I began to think my caro sposo would be absolutely jealous.'

More important social events

Now I must tell you about three more social events which are the background for important developments in the lives of Emma and her friends. First, the much-anticipated ball takes place at the Crown Hotel and is a great success. Emma dances with Frank a lot but feels assured that her heart is safe. She is no longer 'in love' with him and he is making no attempt to raise the temperature of their relationship. Only Harriet has no partner: she is snubbed by Mr Elton, but happily rescued by Mr Knightley, whose humane eagle eye has observed her plight. Afterwards he tells Emma that 'Harriet Smith has some first-rate qualities that Mrs Elton is totally without.'

It is now the middle of June and the weather is fine. Mr Knightley invites everyone to visit his estate at Donwell Abbey and pick some strawberries. The fine old house and its extensive grounds are lovingly described and observed by Emma. The annoying Mrs Elton takes charge of the strawberry picking, chattering away incessantly. Then, as they are getting hot and tired, they retire to the house for a nice cold lunch. We notice that Frank Churchill is, again, mysteriously absent.

Then a rather agitated Jane Fairfax asks Emma to give her apologies because she needs to leave in a hurry. Shortly afterwards, Frank turns up looking hot and bothered and irritable. He tells Emma he is sick of England and is thinking of going abroad. Emma congratulates herself on no longer being in love with 'a man who is so soon discomposed by a hot morning. Harriet's sweet easy temper will not mind it.' So Emma is still matchmaking. But events will soon go rapidly beyond her control.

An expedition to Box Hill

Box Hill is a well-known Surrey beauty spot – you may well have been there yourself. Urged on by Mrs Elton, who hasn't been there, the younger members of the Highbury community agree to a summer outing and a picnic on the hill. Frank is now in a better mood and flirts with Emma in a superficial way. Everyone else is rather subdued, so Frank, in a loud voice, tells them that Emma wants to know what they are all thinking. This doesn't go down too well, so he proposes a different game in which everyone is required to produce 'something entertaining ... either one thing very clever ... or two things moderately clever – or three things very dull indeed ...'. Poor Miss Bates says this is fine for her: 'I shall be sure to say three dull things as soon as I open my mouth, shan't I?'

Quick as a flash, and with surprising cruelty, Emma tells her that her difficulty will be limiting herself to only three dull things. Miss Bates doesn't understand at first, but then catches Emma's meaning and is clearly hurt. The incident seems to be over, but Mr Knightley has seen the whole thing and is very angry with his protégée. He catches up with her as they are getting into the coaches and gives her a terrible ticking off. He points out that Miss Bates fully understood the quip and was really very upset. He goes on to tell her that because Miss Bates is a poor woman who has 'sunk from the comforts she was born to' and has known Emma since she was baby, it is even more reprehensible of Emma to have made her feel ridiculed and humbled. Poor Emma is totally devastated by this major rebuke from the person she respects (and loves?) most in the world and she cries all the way home in the coach.

I'm glad to say that Emma's inner strength and basic good nature rapidly come to the rescue. She goes to see Miss Bates and spends time being thoroughly nice to her. Mr Knightley hears about the visit and Emma is rapidly restored to his good books. He even takes her hand and presses it. Is he going to raise it to his lips? No, he lets it go again.

Spoiler warning: do you want to know the ending?

At this point I should warn anyone who is approaching *Emma* for the first time that we are getting near the end and I am about to make some revelations. So if you really don't want to know what happens in the final chapters *you should stop reading here.*

* * * * * * *

Right, now that they have gone, I can tell you that stunning news stories are about to break with great rapidity in placid little Highbury. First of all, we discover that Frank and Jane have been *secretly engaged for months*! Secrecy seems to have been necessary because of his aunt's disapproval, but she has now conveniently died. This explains why Frank has been coming on to Emma and pretending not to like Jane at all. Diversionary tactics, you see. I'm so glad that Emma wasn't taken in. Once the Frank–Jane romance is in the open Jane perks up wonderfully. She stops looking pale and tired and getting headaches (always ask your tiredness-and-headache patients about their love life) and she and Emma become good friends.

But our heroine now has another problem. For some time, Harriet has been buoyed up by a comment of Emma's to the effect that wonderful things can happen and it is possible for a man to fall in love with and marry a young woman who is socially far beneath him. Emma assumes they have been talking about Frank Churchill, although no names have been mentioned. Now it appears that young Harriet has been nurturing hope about herself and – Mr Knightley! Emma finds herself seriously disturbed by this idea, utterly unreal though it is. 'It darted through her, with the speed of an arrow, that Mr Knightley must marry no one but herself!'

Did you guess that? I wouldn't be surprised. That chemistry was pretty potent from the beginning, but it's fun watching Emma's unconscious feelings rising gradually and then surfacing in a rush. And so, at the end of the book all the tangles are undone and some more attractive knots are tied. Jane Fairfax marries Frank

Churchill; Harriet marries her old love, farmer Robert Martin; and Emma marries Mr Knightley. Their love scenes are very touching: he tells her he has loved her since she was 'thirteen at least' and apologises for all the lecturing: 'I do not believe I did you any good.' (Yes you did, says Emma, affectionately.) She manages to persuade her father that Mr Knightley' s presence at Hartfield as his son-in-law will deter the poultry thieves who have been robbing the neighbours of their 'turkies'. And so everyone in Highbury is happy. Only the Eltons are somewhat miffed. Mr Elton tells his wife he supposes that Emma 'had always meant to catch Knightley if she could'. As for the wedding, Mrs Elton is not at all impressed: 'Very little white satin, very few lace veils; a most pitiful business!' But, of course, we know better. And with that little flourish, like the closing bars of a Mozart opera, Jane Austen rounds off her story. It's a delightful read and you will breathe a deep sigh of satisfaction, mingled with a gentle regret, as your stay in Highbury comes to an end.

The text

Emma by Jane Austen is available in Penguin Classics, with an introduction and notes by Fiona Stafford.

4

Frankenstein

by Mary Shelley (1818)

Gillie Bolton

Words have more power than any one can guess; it is by words that the world's great fight, now in these civilised times, is carried on.

Mary Shelley[1]

Frankenstein concerns what it is to be human. It's about love, power and responsibility: how these forces can lead to ultimate social, political, psychological and spiritual good; and the way power without ethical and moral values and responsibility leads to inhuman degradation and inhumanity. These issues are tackled here on a person-to-person scale; the book is also about the failure of society to take responsibility for people's welfare. A corrupt political and social system will engender corrupt people and social relations.

Frankenstein is a story for our times. It was written by a girl of 19, conceived when she was 17 during a journey around post-French Revolution, war-torn Europe: a time of massive social and political upheaval. It is several stories all wrapped up in each other like an onion, and told in different voices through letters and memories and reports of conversations. Thus we relate to the events and characters from various viewpoints.

The story

Frankenstein is an indulged Swiss lad, brought up in the lap of plenty and shielded from the harshness of life, apart from the death of his beloved mother. He lusts for power, not power over his fellow men, but over the forces of nature. He wishes to overcome death, though nothing could bring back his mother. By long and serious study at the University of Ingoldstadt, he discovers the secret of life, which medicine would love to uncover: that which makes a collection of cells – bone, muscle and organs – a sentient being. But Frankenstein takes no responsibility for his creation. He never feels a pang of guilt, nor takes any responsibility. Frankenstein collects together bits of bodies from charnel houses, dissecting rooms and graveyards. He assembles them into more or less human form, and electrically galvanises his creation into life:

> With an anxiety that almost amounted to agony, I collected the instruments of life around me, that I might infuse a spark of being into the lifeless thing that lay at my feet. It was already one in the morning; the rain pattered dismally against the panes, and my candle was nearly burnt out, when, by the glimmer of the half-extinguished light, I saw the dull yellow eye of the creature open; it breathed hard, and a convulsive motion agitated its limbs.
>
> How can I describe my emotions at this catastrophe, or how delineate the wretch whom with such infinite pains and care I had endeavoured to form? His limbs were in proportion, and I had selected his features as beautiful. Beautiful! – Great God! His yellow skin scarcely covered the work of muscles and arteries beneath; his hair was of a lustrous black, and flowing; his teeth of pearly whiteness; but these luxuriances only formed a more horrid contrast with his watery eyes, that seemed almost of the same colour as the dun-white sockets in which they were set, his shrivelled complexion and straight black lips.
>
> The different accidents of life are not so changeable as the feelings of human nature. I had worked hard for nearly two years, for the sole purpose of infusing life into an inanimate body. For this I had deprived myself of rest and health. I had desired it with an ardour that far exceeded moderation; but now that I had finished, the beauty of the dream vanished, and breathless horror and disgust filled my heart. Unable to endure the aspect of the being I had created, I rushed out of the room. ... (pp 37–8)

And Frankenstein spends the rest of the novel relentlessly pursued by this *fiend*, as he calls him, until the dramatic end.

But our Monster, the anti-hero, says later of himself: 'I was benevolent; my soul glowed with love and humanity' (p 70). Just as Adam and Eve were created by God as guileless and gentle, only eating berries, fruit and seeds, so was the Monster. Like Adam and Eve, he learns of their nakedness and the possibility of sin. He is spurned and attacked by everyone who sees him, even, or especially, by Frankenstein, his creator, his god, or his father – whichever way you want to see it – and the Monster sees it in each of these ways at different times.

The Monster, though created fully grown, has to learn how to live, and what being human is about. He lives in a forest, which is very cold as winter comes on, so when he discovers a little cottage with a lean-to beside it, he is happy. The hovel is inhabited by a French family: blind father, son Felix and daughter. The Monster watches through a crack in the wall between his dwelling and theirs. How they manage to miss seeing such an enormous creature is just one of the mysteries of this text full of delightful improbabilities. He keeps himself secret, having learned that people are terrified and will attack him and run away. He sees his reflection in a pool and realises he is hideous and gigantic, not beautiful like his beloved French family.

The little family are as sad as sad can be, puzzling the Monster, until he realises they are poor, cold and hungry. He plays the 'good spirit', fetching firewood and digging their vegetables from the frozen ground at night. He watches, learns about love and gentleness, and how to speak and communicate. But he has no one with whom to communicate: 'am I not alone, miserably alone?' (p 70). He learns further about their sadness when a beautiful, exotic Muslim stranger appears and stays with them – Felix's lover. The tragedy of their love, estrangement and the loss of the family fortune is one of deceit and treachery. This tale is encapsulated within the main story of Frankenstein and his Creature; but the themes are the same – the transformative nature of love, the potential destructiveness and evil of power and lack of responsibility.

The Monster now learns the power of language – both spoken and written – as Felix instructs his lover in French, enabling him to learn by leaps and bounds when he happens to discover books in the forest. Tragically, he learns even more when he finds Frankenstein's notebooks – that he disgusts and horrifies his creator. He learns about culture and society through reading: an apt model for *Medicine and Literature*. Our Monster is so overwhelmed by his need to be loved that he decides to make himself known to those whom he regards as his own loved ones. He throws himself at the feet of the good, blind old man, who of course offers him what hospitality he can. But when Felix returns and sees this terrifying huge figure clutching at his father's feet, he beats him and chases him away.

The French family all run away from this new terror, unknowing that it is their 'good spirit'. When he realises they are really gone, 'a kind of insanity in my spirits that burst all bounds of reason and reflection' (p 99) overcomes the Monster; he sets fire to their empty cottage and runs away himself. And where does he run to? The only person he has: Frankenstein. But now the knowledge of his abandonment and Frankenstein's disgust has engendered hatred:

> *Unfeeling heartless creator! You had endowed me with perceptions and passions, and then cast me abroad an object for the scorn and horror of mankind. But on you only had I any claim for pity and redress, and from you I determined to seek that justice which I vainly attempted to gain from any other being that wore the human form. My travels were long, and the sufferings I endured intense.* (pp 99–100)

We suffer with the Monster as he is attacked and shot at as he tries to help people. His bitterness increases.

He encounters Frankenstein again only after he has dramatically strangled his beautiful and beloved little brother. Frankenstein catches sight of the Monster in a great flash of lightning – more electricity. They later meet on a glacier on a mountain above Chamonix. The Monster here tells Frankenstein his story since his creation and abandonment – an improbably lengthy and articulately coherent account. He demands that Frankenstein make him a wife, as ugly and horrific as himself. He will take her to an uninhabited part of the world and never trouble Frankenstein again, swearing 'by the blue sky of heaven and by the fire of love that burns in my heart' (p 104). The Monster has realised that his only chance of happiness lies with someone he can love and be loved by. Of course, there is the death of the little boy now as a lever:

> *All men hate the wretched; how, then, must I be hated, who am miserable beyond all living things! Yet you, my creator, detest and spurn me, thy creature to whom thou art bound by ties only dissoluble by the annihilation of one of us. You purpose to kill me. How dare you sport thus with life? Do your duty towards me, and I will do mine towards you and the rest of mankind. ... If you refuse I will glut the maw of death, until it be satiated with the blood of your remaining friends.* (p 69)

Frankenstein, after a horrified deliberation over this ethical dilemma, agrees. Although he returns to his beloved Elizabeth – his adopted cousin and promised wife, and his doting father and best friend, he cannot of course be happy: he has to collect body parts again to make another monster. But he never feels remorse, never takes responsibility for bringing this upon himself and his family by his lust for power over nature: 'I was guiltless' (p 117). The story gets more and more dramatic. Frankenstein goes to Britain with his best friend and retires to the 'desolate and appalling landscape' (p 118) of Orkney for his work of terrible creation. But just as the female Creature is well on the way to completion, he realises he cannot do it. What if she does not want to retire to remote recesses of the globe, what if she is utterly wicked without the first Monster's innate capacity for love? What if, horror of horrors, they procreate? Though why Frankenstein can't use the simple expedient of creating her without the means to do so, Mary Shelley leaves her reader wondering.

As he destroys the half-completed creation, he looks up and there is the Monster at the window with a 'ghastly grin' (p 120). The tables are now turned. The Monster says: 'Slave ... you are my creator, but I am your master; – obey!' Frankenstein will not obey, one of his few moral decisions, so the Monster promises: 'I will be with you on your wedding-night' (p 121). If he can't have sex and love, he is not going to let Frankenstein enjoy them either.

Frankenstein says, 'I was the slave of my creature' (p 110). He had sought to play God in creating life. Now the slave turns slave master. Here follows a Gothic sequence of murder, storms and terror: the best friend is killed, saintly Elizabeth is strangled on her wedding night (in a storm), the father dies, and so on. Frankenstein is pursued by the Monster, just as Aeschylus' Orestes is pursued by the Furies. But Orestes takes full responsibility for killing his mother, the act which brought the Furies down upon him. Eventually Frankenstein is left with no loved ones. Now the pursuer becomes the willingly pursued. Having followed Frankenstein, the Monster now retreats ever northwards, leaving traces so he can be followed but never quite found. We move into a land of mist and snow.

Now I must tell you about the other story. This remarkable book does not have just one stable reliable narrator. The story I have told you so far is partly told by Frankenstein and partly by the Monster himself. But in fact, the whole lot is told by Frankenstein to a ship's captain. Robert Walton is an explorer determined to reach the Pole, another tale of frustrated ambition, another attempt to reach an almost impossible goal. He feels there is something mystical and powerful about the magnetic Pole, and that to get there will give mankind vital and powerful insight. Magnetism was considered as incomprehensible and potentially powerful as electricity at the time of Mary Shelley's writing.

Frankenstein pursues his nemesis, coming across the ice-bound ship of the explorer. He is rescued and tells his tale. Robert Walton writes it down, and that's what we read: the parts of the text in the Monster's voice are quoted by Frankenstein. We also read Robert Walton's letters to his sister about his hopeless voyage. Frankenstein dies and the Monster appears, to the horror of Walton. The Monster is grief-stricken, for this is the death of his father, the only person in the world who has ever had any claim on him:

> My heart was fashioned to be susceptible of love and sympathy; and when wrenched by misery to vice and hatred it did not endure the violence of the change without torture such as you cannot even imagine. ... I was the slave, not the master of an impulse which I detested yet could not disobey ... I cannot believe that I am the same creature whose thoughts were once filled with sublime and transcendent

visions of the beauty and the majesty of goodness. But it is even so; the fallen angel becomes a malignant devil. Yet even that enemy of God and man had friends and associates in his desolation; I am alone. (pp 161–2)

The Monster has the last words in a dramatic, heart-rending speech about abandonment, the effect of the abuse of power and lack of responsibility, and the impossibility of living without love.

The Furies who pursue Orestes for killing his mother, Clytaemnestra, are turned into agents for good and peace by Athene at the end of Aeschylus' *Oresteia*. Frankenstein never learns the lesson, so he never receives absolution as Orestes does. At one point the Monster says to Frankenstein, 'I ought to be thy Adam; but am rather the fallen angel, whom thou drivest from joy for no misdeed. Everywhere I see bliss, from which I alone am irrevocably excluded. I was benevolent and good; misery made me a fiend. Make me happy and I shall again be virtuous' (p 70). Like Adam, the Monster learns a hard lesson, and disaster follows.

We, at the end of this text, see the Monster as a noble creature, a piece of nature ruined by cruelty, lack of love and power with no responsibility. We are all free to make whatever political parallel we like here. I think Mary Shelley would think many of them valid.

Mary Shelley

Mary Shelley was the daughter of the great first feminist, Mary Wollstonecraft, and of the social and politically reformist writer William Godwin, both well-known writers on social equality and justice. Wollstonecraft's *A Vindication of the Rights of Women* was a vital treatise on education and the role of women. Mary's parents believed in the power and responsibility of the individual to effect change. They believed that the inequalities of a culture were mirrored in the familial and private aspects, that the one recapitulates the other. It seems odd, knowing about Mary's mother's great beliefs and works, that Mary created a rather wet, subordinate female character like Elizabeth, and a whole batch of dominant macho men. But *Frankenstein* is powerfully Godwinian in style and ideas.

Wollstonecraft and Godwin did not believe in marriage, but did marry a few months before Mary's birth, to give her legitimacy. Wollstonecraft died of puerperal fever, or a partially retained placenta, when Mary was days old. They did not know then how infection could be carried on the hands of midwives and doctors. Mary was brought up with a strong sense of her clever, wise, deeply principled mother, and a legacy to fulfil. She may well have felt responsible for Wollstonecraft's untimely death. Godwin remarried, but Mary never got on with her step-mother, always missing the mother she never knew.

Mary was well educated, and met many important writers and thinkers. Samuel Taylor Coleridge was a guest, and she and her stepsister hid behind the sofa to hear him recite *The Rime of the Ancient Mariner,* when she was seven or nine. This must have made a huge impact, to judge by this fabulous poem's influence upon *Frankenstein.* There was no television or film of course: only the written and spoken word. Reading aloud and reciting were part of civilised life. Coleridge probably recited with great effect.

Mary may have been struck by the Mariner's psychological need to tell his tale. The Monster similarly recounts his story to Frankenstein very eloquently, and also gives an impassioned speech to Walton immediately after Frankenstein's death. The Monster, like the Ancient Mariner, and like a psychoanalytic patient,[2] seeks therapeutic ease from telling his story and expressing his anger and angst.

Mary wrote from a young age. Her stepsister, Claire, said that they were all expected to be prodigies, especially as writers. Travel is in Mary Shelley's books a metaphor for social, political and individual development, psychologically and spiritually, as in *The Ancient Mariner.* Mary began her literal travelling early, going to the south coast of England for sea bathing to help with a skin condition, and then to Dundee in Scotland at 15. She lived with a happy, stable, deeply Christian family in Dundee and learned to love, particularly their daughter. She also learned to daydream. She began to tell herself stories, and to write them down.

The Walton story in *Frankenstein* possibly started here. Mary heard whaling stories of being locked in the ice, and other dramas of the frozen seas. These must have combined vividly in her mind with the images of *The Ancient Mariner*. She said in her diary that she lived in her imagination in Dundee, having 'waking dreams'.

Mary was born just after the French Revolution, a time of great social and political unrest and change. Among the romantic writers, there was tremendous hope for humanitarian, social and political reform. As Wordsworth wrote: 'Bliss was it in that dawn to be alive / But to be young was very heaven' (*The Prelude*, Book 11).

Mary and Shelley

Percy Bysshe Shelley's turning up in the life of this intense, romantic (in the political sense of the word) 16-year-old, who was much in need of love, was bound to create some stir. Shelley and Mary are both described, at different times, as being 'wild' at this stage. Shelley, although only 21, was married, the father of one child with another on the way. He and Mary consummated their passion in 1813, so the story goes, in St Pancras churchyard, where Wollstonecraft was buried. Shelley, as well as being an ardent Godwinian, would have read Wollstonecraft's writings; they took her travel writing to Europe. Shelley was a passionate romantic, believing in equality and social responsibility. He was also an intellectual; though he didn't prove that at Oxford, being too impetuous and following his own star. He and Mary ran away to war-torn France when she was 16, he 21. They had almost no money, and took with them Mary's stepsister, Claire, who was 15. Claire's mother, Mary's stepmother, followed them fruitlessly as far as Dover. The trio travelled around France, Switzerland and Germany for six weeks (between Napoleon's two campaigns), and returned when they could obtain no more money. They read literature together; the Monster is a self-taught intellectual, just like Mary Shelley herself (except that he has neither her intellectual father nor his wonderful library). She read prodigiously and deeply. Mary and Shelley also wrote a joint journal. Mary was to develop and publish this journal later (travel books were very popular; Mary Wollstonecraft had written one).

They sailed past Castle Frankenstein on the Rhine, and probably heard about Konrad Dippel, the eighteenth-century physician born in the castle who attempted to animate corpses. Mary was expecting her first baby by their return; but it did not long survive its birth. Mary's father and stepmother refused to see them because they weren't married. This, from Godwin, who had not believed in marriage, but then Shelley was already married. His poor wife later killed herself, and Mary and Shelley did marry.

The lovers, still themselves little more than children, were homeless. Claire stayed with them; much to Mary's unhappiness, she was to be with her and Shelley during much of their time together. Whether Claire had a physical relationship with Shelley is not known for certain, but many believed Shelley had sexual relations with both. But Claire fell in love with Byron, which was not clever as Byron was sexually fickle. It left Claire dependent on Shelley, who felt responsible for her; long after his death a chunk of his grandfather's inheritance came to her.

Frankenstein was born while Mary, Shelley and Claire spent time with Byron. The trio travelled to Geneva to stay near Byron's Villa Diodati. Here they read and told ghost stories; Byron recited Coleridge's *Christabel* to dramatic effect. Echoes of *Paradise Lost*, which Shelley read to Mary, are pervasive in *Frankenstein*, and there is evidence of her having read the work of Humphrey Davy, the great experimenter with electricity. There were tremendous electric storms, and they sat around a flickering fire by candlelight trying to frighten each other. It was after one of these sessions that it was suggested they each concoct a terrifying story of their own. Mary had difficulty thinking of one, until she had one of her 'waking dreams'. She was the only one to write hers down, creating one of the best-known novels in the English language.

Frankenstein was Mary's love child, written at the height of Shelley's and her passion. Although she continued to write, it was never with the same vitality. Her novels all convey her inalienable romantic belief in the power of beauty, love and humanitarianism. *Frankenstein* is an inspired text, full of beautiful poetry. Yet it is in many ways immature. The characters are one-dimensional

– Frankenstein himself, for example, makes a brilliant scientific discovery, yet in every other way seems to be rather a dolt; he could be thought to be autistic when he makes no contact with Elizabeth and his family while in Ingoldstadt, but his affection for his friend, Henry Clerval, and his early love for Elizabeth make it clear that he is not. The many improbable coincidences take the text into a fairy-tale land.

Mary's relationship with Shelley soured, possibly due to their endless moving around Europe and Britain, partly to do with always being with other people, particularly Claire, and due to the deaths of their first three children, by the loss of whom Mary was naturally grief-stricken. At the height of their unhappiness, Shelley was drowned on a pleasure trip. By the time Mary was 24 she had travelled extensively in Napoleonic, war-torn Europe, suffered two miscarriages, lost two daughters and a son, and become a widow. She returned to England on the promise of some support for herself and her surviving son, Percy Florence Shelley, from his grandfather, Sir Timothy Shelley. But she was an outcast – recapitulating the fate of the leading characters of her most famous fiction. She remained a marginalised, often reviled member of society, until her death of a brain tumour at 53.

By the time Mary returned to Britain after Shelley's death, the spirit of hope for a just, egalitarian society, with women taking their proper place, was going. It was now a culture turning the corner into Victorian repression and the Industrial Revolution. The old hierarchy was being replaced by one based more on wealth derived from manufacturing, and the powerless masses were now to suffer urban poverty and terrible working conditions and housing. The aspirations of independent-minded women were to be subjugated and crushed by Victorian values. Everything that Mary, the other romantics, and her father and mother had stood for, was disappearing.

The text

Frankenstein, first published on 1 January 1818, has been recreated time and again on stage and screen, very rarely keeping to the spirit of Mary's text. Mary watched the first of these – a farce – in 1823. Because he has no name, the Monster is often called Frankenstein: after all, in *Dracula* the monster is eponymous. The two characters are encountered by many people through film and popular representations, rather than by reading the original texts. This has led to a confusion of the two horrific characters. There is no space here to discuss the relationship between the two, and I will merely say that *Dracula*, in my opinion, is a great romp; it does not offer the moral and ethical questioning and angst of *Frankenstein*.

Mary's reviewers had problems with *Frankenstein*, as with her other novels. Politics and social justice were not supposed to be a woman's sphere, so they were unable to read the social and political messages within her work. *Frankenstein* was first published anonymously, and assumed to be the work of PB Shelley; its readers were shocked to discover it was authored by a woman.

Frankenstein's Monster has been used as a metaphor for terrible things almost since it was first published. The good and noble natural nature of the Monster is invariably forgotten in these comparisons. Lewis Wolpert has called Mary Shelley the wicked stepmother of genetic science; GM crops have been called 'Frankenstein food' – poor Mary and her humanitarian ideals.

Background and associations

Frankenstein is deeply romantic, in the pantheistic as well as the political tradition of Wordsworth and Coleridge. There are many dramatic descriptions of scenery, and a great deal of pathetic fallacy – the Monster is often associated with storms, lightning, and ice grinding and howling. Yet, interestingly, the novel ends not with a bang but a whimper. We don't see the promised dramatic death of the Monster. He leaps from the ship's window and 'He was soon borne away by the waves and lost in darkness and distance.'

The horrid and fearful have probably always fascinated. Perhaps as they sit by their hearths, telling such stories, people make their homes feel more cosy and safe, and the horridness and fear all the more other. A monster set in dramatic scenery is a traditional device. Poor Gawain suffers all sorts of privation from ice, snow, precipices and the like searching for the monstrous Greene Knight, who lives in a dramatically romantic place. The monsters in Beowulf also inhabit gothic environments.

Frankenstein's Monster is hideous and is assumed by all people to be as horrible in thought, spirit and deed, in keeping with Greek and Celtic folk and mythic tradition form. Mary Shelley subverted this in making her monster fundamentally benign. Yet there are now many stories of benevolent monsters – from Oscar Wilde's Selfish Giant to Roald Dahl's Big Friendly Giant. Yet many folk tales relate to care of the poor, needy and possibly monstrously deformed. 'They say the owl was a baker's daughter' (*Hamlet* Act 4, Scene 5, lines 40–41), refers to an old story in which a dirty old beggar asks for bread. The mother starts making him a loaf, but the daughter cuts the dough in half: he does not deserve so much. The beggar is Jesus, and turns her into an owl. Hospitality to a stranger is also vital in Homer: Odysseus returns after his Odyssey incognito as a beggar. Many Postgraduate Education Allowance points might have been earned in heaven, I would have thought, by succouring someone as dreadful as Frankenstein's Monster.

The Monster is never named, but always Monster, Fiend or Creature – never human, never accorded personhood. This is his enduring grief and tragedy: he has all the fine feelings of a person, and the ability to learn and reason and develop his understanding, but this is never recognised. Naming is a powerful process: in many cultures, the naming ceremony is a vital rite of passage. Babies were once considered unable to go to heaven until baptised and christened. In the final section, the Monster calls Frankenstein 'Man', un-naming him, and making him stand for all mankind, just as the Monster himself stands for all the unnamed wronged of the earth.

The word 'slave' is used of both Frankenstein and the Monster. Slaves were not thought human any more than the Monster. It has been considered that Mary Shelley might have intended *Frankenstein* as an anti-slavery text. She encountered the slave trade in Bristol and perhaps modelled her monster, in part, on

African slaves. Slaves were often not called by their own name by their masters, who gave them easier names. This was also often true of Victorian mistresses: maids might always be called Betsy, whatever their real names. The servant was that much less human than her mistress.

Frankenstein has also been considered to be about the French Revolution, the monster being the Jacobite mob. As such, it has been thought to be anti-revolutionary. I feel sure the ethics, ethos and spirit of the revolution are represented by the text, and it seems a simplification to think that the Monster might just stand for the mob. Frankenstein partly also grew out of the horrific practice of body-snatching, that is the taking of bodies from burial grounds for dissection for medical education.

Frankenstein is also about parenting. Mary's mother died when she was days old, and her own baby died while she was writing. Frankenstein had wonderful parents – good, kind, loving and supportive. But, although he is deeply affected by the death of his mother, this does not explain why he rejects his own 'child', immediately it comes to life. He takes no responsibility, offering it neither love nor care.

A lack of strong, enduring and developmental love relationships in childhood possibly leads to violence in adulthood. I think this is partly why our hearts go out to the Monster, despite his terrible deeds. The theme of the nobility of friendship is also important in *Frankenstein*. The ship's captain, Walton, longs for a male soul mate and feels he may have found one in Frankenstein at the end of the story; Frankenstein's bosom friend, Clerval, is always vitally important to him; Felix honourably befriends his lover's father (who then betrays him); and Elizabeth is heartbroken when her loyal servant and friend is executed wrongly for the murder of the little boy. How much must Mary Shelley have longed for a proper friend, having never had a mother, and enduring a poisonous relationship with Claire, her stepsister. She was later much disappointed in her women friends, on whom she tended to rely, and in whom she tended to trust, too much.

Frankenstein was written in the same period as the restrained and cultured novels of Jane Austen. Gothic novels had already come into fashion: Austen's *Northanger Abbey* is a spoof. Some of our best-known horrific characters followed on from *Frankenstein*, for example in: *Dracula* (Bram Stoker), *Dr Jekyll and Mr Hyde* (RL Stephenson) and *The Portrait of Dorian Grey* (Oscar Wilde).

Why read *Frankenstein*?

Mary Shelley's subtitle is *The Modern Prometheus*: Frankenstein discovers the mystery of life, just as Prometheus did, according to some classical accounts. But she is very reticent about how the Monster is created: there's no science in this book, no recipe for the reader to create their own tame monster. She also doesn't explain why the bits of which the Monster is made don't decompose while Frankenstein is collecting them.

No medical or healthcare practitioner would ever be presented with a patient such as the Monster, thankfully. But the Monster and his maker are metaphors for all sorts of things, not least a range of patients. The Monster perhaps only exists in the mind of a schizophrenic, personality disordered or paranoid Frankenstein, power mad with an innate lack of responsibility. The Monster is seriously deformed and disabled in body, though not in spirit and mind; once persecuted he becomes manic depressive, perhaps. Medicine has come no nearer, and probably never will, to understanding what it is that a dead body has lost, what that animating spark is. Recognising this non-understanding, and the wonderful mystery, could help greater acceptance of death, which is too readily seen as a medical failure. Old people could perhaps be considered to be noble, and old age respected, rather than being seen as merely a frightening stage on the way to death.

Mary Shelley offers a warning to scientific research with *Frankenstein*, which resonates with current fears about nanotechnology and genetic research. She debunks the positivist notion of progress, warning how destructive scientific progress can be without moral responsibility. We only have to look to nuclear research to know this. Adam and Eve were perfectly happy in their ignorance and their undeveloped society; we are not perfectly happy in our 'civilised' culture. Mary Shelley presents a noble savage, reworking the old story that we are all born good and equal and free, until we experience the destructiveness of the inhumanity of man to man. Frankenstein himself was also noble and good in the pre-Ingoldstadt days before he came into contact with research and the idea of scientific progress; Walton calls him noble in the end, a ruined piece of nature like his Monster.

The eighteenth-century surgeon anatomist William Hunter urged his students to gain a 'necessary inhumanity' by dissecting the dead. 'Clinical detachment' is a more modern expression.[3] Frankenstein becomes inhumane through dissection and resection, cutting himself off from family and friends. Dissection, if carefully handled, does not of course dehumanise people; but many medical education and training experiences can have this tendency. The study of medical humanities, including literature, as an integral element of medical (pre- and post-experience) education can help to prevent this happening.[4]

Medicine and healthcare are about care, nurture, power, ethics, moral and human values, responsibility and love; just as *Frankenstein* is. That's really why I want you to read it. Mary Shelley, with her masterpiece of human suffering, wields the power of words to transform the experience of her readers – you and me.

The text

Shelley M (1993) *Frankenstein or the Modern Prometheus*. Wordsworth Editions, Hertfordshire. (All page references in this chapter are to the Wordsworth edition.)

References

1   Bennett BT (1996) *Novels and Selected Work of Mary Shelley*, vol 6, p 213. Pickering & Chatto, Baltimore.

2   Brewer WD (1994) Mary Shelley on the therapeutic value of language. *Papers on Language and Literature* **30**(4): 387–407.

3   Richardson R (2000) 'A necessary inhumanity?' *Journal of Medical Ethics: Medical Humanities* **26**: 104–6.

4 Bolton G (2003) Medicine, the arts and humanities. *Lancet* **362**: 93–4.

Further reading

- Bennett BT (1998) *Mary Shelley: an introduction*. Johns Hopkins University Press, Baltimore.

- Garrett M (undated) *Mary Shelley*. The British Library, London.

- Seymour M (2000) *Mary Shelley*. John Murray, London.

5

Jane Eyre

by Charlotte Brontë (1847)

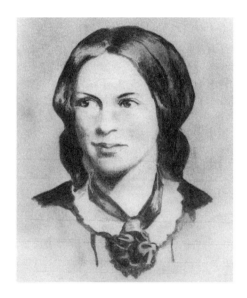

On Wednesday 15 August 1846, Charlotte Brontë took her almost blind father from Haworth to Manchester to consult a highly recommended eye surgeon, Mr WJ Wilson. On the following Monday, Mr Wilson removed the cataract from Patrick Brontë's left eye. The operation lasted 15 minutes and was performed without an anaesthetic. He recorded the experience in the margins of his copy of Graham's *Modern Domestic Medicine*: 'the feeling … under the operation was of a burning nature – but not intolerable'. When it was over he had to lie in a darkened room with bandages over his eyes most of the time for four weeks. He was also bled with leeches from the temples. But the operation was a success and when the bandages were finally removed he could see again with his left eye. Meanwhile, in her Manchester lodgings, Charlotte was writing furiously in pencil in her little square notebooks. She was working on the first draft of her second novel: *Jane Eyre*.

On 15 July 1847, she parcelled up the complete manuscript and popped it in the post to Messrs Smith, Elder and Co., publishers, of Cornhill, London. At that stage she and her sisters were pretending to be three brothers called Bell, because they thought that publishers would be prejudiced against unknown women writers. Smith, Elder had not been very impressed with her first book (*The Professor*), although they could see evidence of talent, and they encouraged Mr Bell to keep writing. But *Jane Eyre* totally blew them away. The head of the firm, George Smith, spent a whole Sunday reading it and enthusiastically accepted it for publication. Since then *Jane Eyre* has remained a bestseller and may even be the most widely read novel in the world.

Why was it so special? And why has it remained irresistible even to hard-bitten modern readers? Well, it's the story of a young girl's triumph over adversity, which is a pretty good basis for any novel. But it was also the first novel ever in which a child seems to be telling her own story. Jane Austen's *Mansfield Park* (1816) also has a little orphan as a heroine, but the narrator is the author. Dickens' *David Copperfield* did not appear until two years after *Jane Eyre*. And furthermore, Charlotte Brontë's heroine is a fierce little fighter who is not afraid of telling the grown-ups what she thinks of them when she is only 10. Later on, she has a passionate affair with a romantic older man, breaks her heart, suffers, nearly makes the wrong decision and finally wins through. You probably read it and loved it in your teens (especially if you were a girl), but your recollection is now hazy. If you haven't read it you have such a treat in store. So sit back and prepare to enjoy while I tell you all about it.

The story begins

'There was no possibility of taking a walk that day.' With that opening sentence we are plunged straight into the world of Gateshead Hall, Jane's first home. There are three other children in the room but they are 'clustered round their Mama', who is lying on the sofa. She has ordered Jane to remain at a distance until she can be better behaved. So Jane retreats to the breakfast room to take comfort in a book about birds that inhabit chilly, inhospitable Arctic landscapes. Gradually we realise what is going on in this house. Jane is 10 years old. She is being reluctantly fostered by her aunt, Mrs Reed, who treats her with none of the affection she lavishes on her own three children. The two girls, though spoilt and unfriendly, are just about bearable, but 14-year-old John, 'large and stout for his age, with a dingy and unwholesome skin', is a real bully. When he spies Jane reading quietly, he orders her to stand before him and hits her 'for your impudence in answering Mamma a while since' and calls her a rat. He then takes her book and throws it at her. She falls down and cuts her head. But our little heroine has plenty of courage: 'Wicked and cruel boy!' she says, 'You are like a a murderer – you are a slave driver – you are like the Roman Emperors!' John attacks her, there is a scuffle, and when they are separated by the housemaids, Jane the outsider is accused of assaulting John. 'Take her away to the red-room and lock her in there,' says the terrible Mrs Reed.

In the red-room

By now, our hearts are palpitating in time with Jane's. We are absolutely with her, there is no escape. What on earth is going to happen to us in the red-room? It sounds really frightening. But before we get there, Jane's status is made even clearer to us. The two maids, Bessie and Abbot, struggle to hold her down and Abbot tells her that she is 'less than a servant, for you do nothing for your keep'. She must on no account think that she has equal status with the Reed children, she must be humbly grateful that she has not been consigned to the poorhouse. Then they bundle her into the red-room and shut the door. The decoration of the red-room is pretty much red, although the pillows and counter-pane of the large (red-curtained) bed are snowy white. This is the bed in which the late Mr John Reed, Jane's benevolent uncle, breathed his last. Before his death, Uncle Reed had made his wife promise to bring Jane up as one of her own children. But although he was a decent chap in life, the room where he expired is chilly and spooky. Will his ghost return to haunt it as darkness falls and the wind howls outside? Jane is still boiling with rage and resent-ment, but she is also fearful. She is only 10 for goodness sake. Suddenly a streak of light moves up the wall and across the ceiling. Jane panics and starts to scream. Mrs Reed and the maids come flying. But they dismiss her screams as mere naughtiness and lock her in again. She has 'some sort of fit' and loses consciousness.

The next day, Jane wakes up in her own bed in the nursery. The doctor has been called. Well, actually, it's the apothecary, Mr Lloyd, 'sometimes called in by Mrs Reed when the servants were ailing: for herself and the children she employed a physician'. I am sure you are aware that the apothecary was the GP of the day; so now we are placed well and truly on Jane's side of the social divide. And who would wish to be anywhere else? Mr Lloyd is quite a good fellow, I'm happy to say. Although he is a little slow to grasp the nature of his little patient's situation, he does at least listen to her and allow her to contradict his naïve impression that she is enjoying a happy family life with the Reeds. 'Has she no other relations?', asks Mr Lloyd. Well, she might have some poor ones on her father's side, says Jane, but she wouldn't want to go to them. She has seen poor children begging and she doesn't want to be one of them (sensible girl). The only other option seems to be to go to school. This idea appeals to Aunt Reed too. She is only too pleased to find a way of getting rid of her rebellious and ungrateful niece.

Jane confronts Mr Brocklehurst

A few weeks later, Jane is summoned to the breakfast room to meet a tall, grim clergyman called Mr Brocklehurst. His body looks to her like a black stone pillar and 'the grim face at the top was like a carved mask, laced above the shaft by way of a capital'. 'Well, Jane Eyre, and are you a good child?' he enquires. Mrs Reed shakes her head and adds 'perhaps the less said about that the better, Mr Brocklehurst'.

And so Jane's interrogation begins. It makes compulsive reading because she is quite a tough little kid and is not to be totally squashed. When the black pillar asks where the wicked go after death she tells him: 'They go to hell', and she knows that hell is a pit of fire. But when he asks what she must do to avoid falling into the pit her reply is: 'I must keep in good health and not die.' Mr Brocklehurst coldly tells her that children younger than Jane die daily. They then have a conversation about the Bible and when Jane says she doesn't find the psalms interesting, Mr Brocklehurst tells her, 'That proves you to have a wicked heart.' Then Mrs Reed goes on about Jane having 'a tendency to deceit'. Mr Brocklehurst is shocked but is confident that his methods will take care of Jane's character problems. Arrangements are clearly being made to send her away to Mr Brocklehurst's school where she will be taught to be humble and useful in accordance with her aunt's wishes. As a parting gift Mr Brocklehurst offers her a book called the *Child's Guide*, containing 'an account of the awfully sudden death of Martha G—, a naughty child addicted to falsehood and deceit'.

When he has gone, Jane, who is absolutely on fire with the injustice that she has suffered, turns on Mrs Reed with a passionate speech of rebuttal. 'I am not deceitful: if I were I would say I loved *you*; but I declare I do not love you; I dislike you the worst of anybody in the world except John Reed: and this book about the Liar you may give to your girl Georgiana, for it is she who tells lies and not I.' She ends her tirade by telling her aunt: 'People think you are a good woman but you are bad, hard hearted. *You* are deceitful!'

Mrs Reed is quite shaken, and Jane experiences a new sense of freedom and triumph. But soon she will be sent away to That School.

The first form at Lowood

At five the next morning Jane is up and dressed, says goodbye to Bessie (who has been kind to her) and is carried off by the coach on a 50-mile journey to Lowood School. Charlotte Brontë modelled Lowood on the school 'for the daughters of clergy' at Cowan Bridge, in a remote part of the Yorkshire Pennines, to which four of the Brontë sisters were dispatched because their father could afford nothing better. I am not sure how bad Cowan Bridge was, but Lowood is probably the scariest school in English literature. If I had to choose, I think I would rather be educated at Dotheboys Hall.

We are given a detailed account of Jane's first night and day at Lowood. We see the long schoolroom during the evening prep session. Eighty girls of ages ranging from 9 or 10 to 20 are seated on benches at four deal tables. What are they whispering? They are trying to learn their lessons by heart ready for tomorrow. The dormitory is another long room where the girls sleep two to a bed. In the morning they have prayers and Bible reading for at least an hour before breakfast. At last, it's time for breakfast and the girls are served with the famous Lowood burnt porridge, which no one can eat. The rest of the day consists of what sound like very dreary lessons punctuated by bells, shouted orders and more disgusting food. However, the oppressive atmosphere is lightened a little by the presence of the superintendent, Miss Temple, who is beautiful and dignified and admired by all. It is Miss Temple who orders a special extra meal of bread and cheese to make up for the inedible porridge.

Helen Burns and Miss Scatcherd: the reign of terror

During a welcome break, Jane wanders out into the garden and meets 13-year-old Helen Burns, who will become her best friend. Later in the afternoon, Helen is made to stand in the middle of the room as punishment for some unnamed offence. This discipline is inflicted by Miss Scatcherd, whose very name is enough to strike fear and trembling into all of us as we cower behind our books and hope that she won't notice us. Miss Scatcherd has really got it in for Helen. On the second day she berates her for having dirty fingernails. No one has been able to wash because the water in the pitchers was frozen. A little later on, to Jane's horror (and ours) Helen has to fetch a nasty bundle of twigs with which Miss Scatcherd whips her on her bare neck. Helen bears it with fortitude. Her problem, as she tells Jane later, is that she can't help being untidy and scruffy. Or as Miss Scatcherd would put it, 'slatternly'. But Helen doesn't harbour her tormentor or anyone else any grudges. She has her own creed, she tells Jane 'which no-one ever taught me'. Helen believes that there is no point in brooding on injustice; nobody is perfect and it's much better to forgive those who wrong you and wait patiently for the world to come, which 'extends hope to all'. Jane is deeply impressed, but of course this kind of noble submission is impossible for her. Thank goodness.

The inspector calls

Life at Lowood continues through the winter. Like everyone else, Jane is cold and hungry and bored. Sundays are particularly bad with a two-hour walk to church and an even colder walk back in the evening after two services. After three weeks have passed, Mr Brocklehurst makes his first appearance to carry out an inspection. He admonishes Miss Temple for having given the girls an extra meal. 'Oh, madam, when you put bread and cheese, instead of burnt porridge into these children's mouths, you may indeed feed their vile bodies, but you little think how you starve their immortal souls!' This is the Brocklehurst version of evangelical Christianity. His next stroke of genius is to decide that the girls' hair is too long and all their 'topknots' must be cut off. Just then his wife and daughters appear, expensively dressed, with ostrich feathers decorating their fashionable hats, and lovely long hair 'elaborately curled'. Charlotte is really piling on the savage irony here. But worse is to come. Jane, in her nervous state, drops a slate and draws attention to herself. The black marble clergyman recognises her. He makes her stand on a stool and informs the assembled school that Jane is a servant and agent of the Evil one, and, of course, a Liar! The female Brocklehursts are deeply shocked and poor Jane has to stand there for the rest of the day with this public condemnation ringing in her ears.

Tea and typhus

That evening, Helen comforts Jane by pointing out that none of the girls thinks any the less of her because she has been picked on by Mr Brocklehurst, who is universally disliked. Later on, kind Miss Temple comes to her aid and Jane tells her the story of her sufferings in the Reed household and Mrs Reed's false accusation of deceit. Miss Temple makes it clear that she doesn't believe these calumnies and gives her a motherly kiss. Then she invites Helen and Jane for tea in her room. They each have 'a delicious but thin morsel of toast' followed by a generous slice of 'a good-sized seed cake'. Can life at Lowood really be about to improve? Well, yes and no. The next day, Helen is made to wear a piece of pasteboard with the word 'slattern' on her forehead for not tidying up her things properly. Yes, Miss Scatcherd again. In a modern school story that woman would meet a grisly death. But sad to say it is the poor little girls of Lowood who start to die. There is an outbreak of typhus at the school and their undernourished bodies are in no state to withstand it. Forty-five of the 80 girls fall ill. Some go home to die; others perish at school and are hastily buried. Unhappily, our good friend Helen is one of the victims. Jane is with her on her deathbed, where she lies exhausted by fits of coughing but with her simple Christian faith undiminished.

Eventually Jane falls asleep with her arms round her friend's neck and wakes to find her dead. This scene could well have been sentimental. But it is firmly based on Charlotte's own experience and so well written that it can still bring tears. Helen was modelled on Charlotte's beloved eldest sister, Maria, who had taken care of her at Cowan Bridge School. Both Maria and the next oldest sister, Elizabeth, were brought home from Cowan Bridge to die.

A new beginning

You may have observed that life at school tends to improve once you get into the sixth form. Maybe as you grew up you were better able to cope with it, maybe you were treated better, or perhaps the school just got better. We now find Jane looking back on eight years at Lowood – six as a pupil and a further two years as a teacher. It seems that after the typhus terror had receded, Lowood acquired more funding and better management (Mr Brocklehurst was sidelined) and rose rapidly in the league table of Yorkshire schools.

Our heroine now presents herself to us as a well-educated young woman of 18, looking forward to making her way in the world. Unfortunately, the only career open to her is that of tutor to the children of a wealthy family: or in other words the profession of governess, hated and despised by all nineteenth-century women writers. Jane applies for a situation and secures a job at Thornfield, a country house 70 miles south of Lowood and therefore approximately in the Midlands. Arriving at night, Jane is welcomed by the housekeeper, Mrs Fairfax, and given a tour of the house, which is a substantial manor with battlements. She is glad to have a cosy bedroom of her own after her years as a dependant. In the morning, after getting dressed, she considers her appearance: 'I sometimes wished to have rosy cheeks, a straight nose and a cherry mouth: I desired to be tall, stately and finely developed in figure; I felt it a misfortune that I was so little, so pale and had features so irregular and so marked.' However, she is quite pleased with her little black Quaker dress and clean white tucker.

It is unusual for our Jane to bother about her appearance. Is she hoping to meet someone special in her new life? She is introduced to her pupil, a little French girl called Adèle, who is the ward of her new employer, Mr Rochester. Adèle is cute, friendly and artistic, if not a very dedicated student. There is no sign yet of Mr Rochester, whose visits, although rare, are, according to Mrs Fairfax, 'always sudden and unexpected'.

Another slightly odd thing I should tell you about Thornfield Hall is that on Jane's first day, as she is returning from inspecting the view from the roof, she hears a strange peal of laughter coming from a bedroom on the third floor. 'It was a curious laugh – distinct, formal, mirthless.' The laughing one appears to be a stout servant called Grace Poole. Mrs Fairfax, the housekeeper, just tells her to be quiet. So can we now forget all about it? I don't think so.

First meeting with the master

Nevertheless, Jane seems to be enjoying her new home and her new job. Three months later, on a beautiful January afternoon, she sets off down the lane on a two-mile walk to post a letter. As the sun sets she sits on a stile and looks back at the battlements of Thornfield. Suddenly she hears the thunder of hoof beats as a horse and rider gallop towards her. Then the horse slips and falls on a sheet of ice. Jane runs to the rescue. Who is the mysterious fallen horseman? It is of course Mr Rochester himself, the glamorous but dangerous older man whom you may remember from previous readings of *Jane Eyre*. When he struggles to his feet we can take a look at him (in the moonlight). He is of middle height with 'considerable breadth of chest'. 'He had a dark face, with stern features and a heavy brow … he was past youth, but had not yet reached middle age; perhaps he might be thirty-five.'

The lord and master has sprained his ankle and Jane has to help him back onto his horse. Always a bit of a tease, he elicits from her that she is the governess at Thornfield Hall but doesn't let on that he is the boss. Only when she gets back to the house does she hear that Mr Rochester is now in residence.

Jane and Rochester: the relationship develops

We now follow the fascinating development of Jane's relationship with Edward Rochester. As I am sure you knew, or have guessed by now, he is going to become the love in Jane's life. But he is by no means a conventional Prince Charming. For one thing he is so old! Not that I have anything against older men: Jane Austen's Mr Knightley comes favourably to mind as an example, but he is better dressed, utterly reliable and has perfect manners. In other words, he is cool, which Mr Rochester definitely is not. Furthermore Mr Rochester has a very murky past, as we shall soon discover. In their first formal interview he interrogates Jane in a rough but sympathetic way about her background and her childhood. He wants to hear her play the piano and asks to see her drawings. He gives credit where it is due, but he doesn't go in for fulsome praise. Then he disappears for a few more weeks. When they next meet, they have one of those important conversations in which people really get to know each other. She always gives him straight answers to his impertinent questions; when asked if she thinks him handsome, she simply says 'No, sir'. She doesn't think he is a fool, but she has the nerve to enquire if he is a philanthropist. He complains about 'another stick of the pen-knife', but her frankness allows him to reflect on his feelings about his past life and his mistakes. Their conversation combines bluntness and a certain amount of mutual teasing, which is great fun to read. He is the stern, autocratic master who is ashamed of his past; she is the timid little governess who is not afraid to correct his morals. There is no talk of love at this stage, but it is intimate and erotic nonetheless.

Jane and Rochester continue to meet and talk whenever he summons her to his presence in the evenings. He tells her about his affair with a French dancer, which led to his adopting her daughter (although he claims not to be the father). At least we now know where Jane's little pupil, Adèle, fits into the picture. Jane forgives him for his past sins (without condoning them) and their relationship seems to have taken another big step forward. But she can't help noticing his moodiness and harsh way of talking to the servants. Sometimes he gives Jane a black scowl too. What is troubling him? Why does he keep going away? In the night Jane is woken by a repetition of that horrible laughter, followed by a gurgling and moaning. She goes out to investigate and finds smoke pouring from Mr Rochester's room. His bed curtains are on fire and he is still asleep! Resourceful Jane puts out the fire with a well-aimed jug of water, waking the master in the process and saving his life. Has Grace Poole, the mad servant woman, been responsible? He won't say, but he doesn't want Jane to go. He starts to tell her that she has struck delight into his innermost heart. No one else is awake. Will they spend the night together? No way. This is a Victorian novel, so Jane goes back to her own room, but she doesn't sleep: 'Till morning dawned I was tossed on a buoyant but unquiet sea, where billows of trouble rolled under surges of joy.'

A rival appears

Will Jane and Rochester get married? What will be done about Grace Poole and why is her eccentric, not to say dangerous, behaviour treated with such toleration? We shall find out in good time, but first I must briefly describe some of the subsequent events at Thornfield. For a while, Jane appears to have a serious rival in the elegant shape of Miss Blanche Ingram, the daughter of a neighbouring landowner. Mr Rochester even gives everyone to understand that they are engaged and he seriously intends to marry her. Jane is cruelly disappointed but seems to resign herself to the inevitable. She is, after all, very plain compared with Miss Ingram and she is only a governess. Rochester throws a magnificent house party, the like of which Thornfield has rarely seen. All the local gentry and their families are invited, including of course his fiancée. Jane is invited to join in but as the governess, remains an invisible non-person to all these posh visitors. They play charades, and Jane has to go through the pain of watching Rochester and Blanche playing the parts of bride and groom. (I hear echoes of the play-acting in *Mansfield Park*, but Charlotte never read any Jane Austen until after *Jane Eyre* was published and was not impressed when she did.) Poor Jane: she has learned to love Mr Rochester, how can she 'unlove him now', she wonders, 'merely because I found that he had ceased to notice me'.

But Mr Rochester is still teasing. He even gets himself up in female drag and passes himself off as an itinerant fortune-teller who offers to read the palms of all the ladies. Jane is persuaded to have a consultation too, and the old crone accurately portrays her character. 'Chance has meted out to you a measure of happiness,' he tells her. She has only to stretch out her hand and take it up. This is the strangest and perhaps the least-reported chapter in *Jane Eyre*. When he has removed his disguise and been gently reproved by his client, she tells him that a visitor from the West Indies called Mr Mason has arrived. This sends Rochester into shock. Jane doesn't know what is the matter or how she can help.

More alarms at night

That very night there is a major disturbance. Jane hears a loud cry followed by the sounds of a struggle on the third floor (Grace Poole's territory). The assault has taken place in what appears to be a secret room, leading off from inside one of the third-floor bedrooms, the inner door screened by a tapestry. In here they find Mr Mason, bleeding from the arm and shoulder. Someone has savagely attacked him with a knife. And also teeth. There is no sign of Grace Poole but Jane assumes that she is the perpetrator. Once again, the incident is smoothed over without an explanation. But Mr Rochester is clearly struggling with himself over something to do with Jane. He keeps asking her whether a man could be forgiven for overstepping the rules of conduct and propriety, if the attainment of a better life depended on it. What dark secret is he keeping back? It's about Grace Poole, isn't it? Have you guessed? For the present, he is not going to reveal it, and reverting to teasing mode, he goes back to telling Jane about his fiancée, whom he describes as 'a real strapper, Jane: big, brown, and buxom'. He makes her sound like a horse, but Jane is still pretty upset.

Love at last

Mr Rochester at first continues to maintain that he is going to marry Blanche and that he has arranged for Jane 'to undertake the education of the five daughters of Mrs Dionysius O'Gall of Bitternut Lodge, Connaught, Ireland'. This is so far away that she is unlikely to see her friend and master again. Jane is distraught.

Finally Rochester drops the teasing and tells her that he loves her and that she, Jane, is the only girl he intends to marry. At first she can't believe it. But it's true, he means it. That night there is a terrific thunderstorm and the great horse chestnut tree at the bottom of the orchard is struck by lightning and split in two. Someone or something seems to be registering an objection.

Another ghastly night at Thornfield

The chestnut tree notwithstanding, preparations for the wedding go forward. Edward tries to deck his bride-to-be in jewels and finery but she prefers to remain dressed as the governess. Then, while Rochester is away, Jane has a series of nightmares. In the first two she has to carry a wailing child (perhaps her child self). In the third and most fearful one, a strange woman with a ghastly purple face and bloodshot eyes appears in her bedroom. The apparition removes Jane's wedding veil from the closet and puts it on her own head. 'Then it removed my veil from its gaunt head, rent it in two parts, and flinging both parts on the floor, trampled on them.' But the really creepy part is that in the morning she finds the veil really is lying on the carpet, torn in two. Just as the tree was split in two by lightning.

Spoiler warning

At this point if you don't want me to give away the rest of the plot you had better stop reading. Those of you who don't care, or have guessed the meaning of the night visitation, or knew anyway, may stay with me. I hope that you do, because *Jane Eyre* is a classic, which means that however many times you read it, the twists and turns of the plot retain their ability to surprise and excite because of the sheer quality of the writing.

The next sensational event is that the wedding ceremony is interrupted by a solicitor from London, who says he has proof *that Mr Rochester is already married and that his wife is alive.* The witness is Mr Mason, the knife victim, who is the lady's brother.

Now at last, Mr Rochester has to reveal his terrible secret. He leads everyone to the secret room on the third floor and introduces Mrs Rochester. She is a shaggy-haired, purple-faced, growling monster of a woman, whom Jane recognises as the woman who tore up her veil. Yes, Mr Rochester is married to a mad woman (called Bertha) whom he has kept locked up in his house for years. Grace Poole is merely the dedicated servant who has the job of looking after her. Mrs Rochester tries to attack her husband and has to be forcibly restrained. It's all very upsetting and I feel very sorry for both him and Jane.

In the ensuing chapters he tries desperately to persuade Jane to live with him anyway; but of course her Lowood training reasserts itself and she refuses. Although it breaks her poor little heart to do so, she resolves to leave Rochester and Thornfield at once.

Rochester's mad wife is an intriguing mystery. Since it is never safe to go near her, we never really get to know her as a person. The writer Jean Rhys tried to reconstruct Bertha's early life and marriage to Rochester in the West Indies in a novel called *Wide Sargasso Sea*. However, Sandra Gilbert and Susan Gubar have suggested in their book *The Madwoman in the Attic* that Bertha is psychologically a part of Jane herself. The madwoman can be seen as a kind of projection of some of our little heroine's own violent and out-of-control feelings. If this seems alarming, consider that as a child Jane also found herself locked up (in the red-room) because her rage (and perhaps her jealousy of her cousins) seemed to be uncontainable. And it is interesting to remember that Charlotte Brontë was once herself hopelessly in love with a married man. His name was M. Heger, who was her teacher during her stay in Brussels, and his wife was perfectly sane. We don't know if Heger returned her feelings, but nothing much seems to have happened, although Charlotte may have suffered torments of jealousy which she had to lock up in the secret room at Thornfield.

Escape to Moor House

Jane bundles up some belongings and sneaks out of Thornfield at dawn. She walks to the nearest town, spends all her money and takes the coach for as long a ride as she can afford. She is deposited at a crossroads and then just carries on walking. She reaches a village and tries to find work, but there isn't any. She's hungry; she tries to barter her handkerchief for a bread roll but the village shopkeeper is not interested. She is reduced to begging for bread and, at her lowest point, eagerly accepting in her hand some porridge that a little girl was about to throw out to the pigs. That reminds me of the horrible burnt porridge on her first day at Lowood. She staggers on over fields and moors and a marsh. She is very nearly dead from starvation, exhaustion and exposure. Finally, she reaches a house where she begs to be admitted for shelter. The servant is unwilling to let this scarecrow figure through the kitchen door at first. Then, when all seems lost, the man of the house arrives and shows Jane some Christian hospitality.

Jane has happily and completely fortuitously arrived at the house of the two Rivers sisters, Diana and Mary, and their clergyman brother, the Reverend St John Rivers. She is given some bread and milk and a bed for the night, but is too tired to tell them anything about herself until she has slept. In the morning, Mr Rivers, a tall, slim young man of about 28–30, elicits Jane's story. She tells him and his sisters that she is the orphan daughter of a clergyman, but she pretends her name is Jane Elliot. She tells them about Lowood and Mr Brocklehurst. By the time she is halfway through, they can all see that she is thoroughly respectable and that they did right to let her stay. Furthermore, Mr Rivers is inclined to find her a job as a teacher.

Moor House (as it is called) proves to be a good place in which to recuperate and take stock. It's situated in beautiful country: there are pasture fields with sheep and 'their little mossy faced lambs' and purple moors in the distance. We are clearly back in North Yorkshire or perhaps even Cumbria. And, best of all, Jane gets on very well with Diana and Mary; it's like having two really nice sisters who share your taste in reading and drawing. But soon it is time to move on. The Rivers family are short of cash as their uncle has disinherited them. Mary and Diana must go south to become governesses (oh no!) and St John will be moving to the vicarage in the village of Morton, with Hannah, the servant. Jane agrees to go with them to supervise the new Morton school for village girls. She has a nice cottage to live in, her pupils are moderately willing to learn and give no trouble. Jane feels she ought to be happy. But, not surprisingly, she still finds herself weeping over the loss of Mr Rochester.

A man with a mission

I don't need to remind you that there is now a younger and more eligible man in the vicinity. As with Mr Rochester, there is already a beautiful rival for his affections, called Rosamond Oliver. St John confesses to Jane that he loves Rosamond and he thinks she likes him. But, alas, they can never be married because he intends to leave England to work as a missionary in the East and Rosamond would be totally unsuited to this sort of life. Jane suggests, innocently, that if he really loves Rosamond he might 'relinquish the scheme' to become a missionary. St John is shocked. 'Relinquish! What! My vocation? My great work? My foundation laid on earth for a mansion in heaven?' St John hopes to be numbered in the select band of people whose evangelical works will guarantee them a place in heaven. His resolve is firm. He is not a man of flesh, he tells Jane. His soul is 'just as fixed as a rock, firm set in the depths of a restless sea. Know me to be what I am – a cold, hard man.' He is so cold and hard that many critics have seen him as a sort of equivalent of Mr Brocklehurst, carved in white stone rather than black. He also has an icy quality, which contrasts vividly with Jane's temperament of fire.

Now there are some rapid developments in the plot. St John turns up at Jane's little cottage one snowy morning in January and tells her that he has discovered all about her real history. How has he found out? It seems that Mr Briggs, the solicitor who interrupted the wedding, has been searching for Jane because she has come into some money. We are astonished to learn that the Rivers family are Jane's cousins (their father was her mother's brother) and their Uncle John in the West Indies has just died and left Jane £20,000. Jane thinks it's unfair of him to leave out his Rivers nephew and nieces, and she insists on splitting the money with them so that they have £5000 each.

Will Jane succumb?

Now St John begins his campaign to get Jane to come to India with him. He can see that, unlike Rosamond, Jane would be an ideal missionary's wife because of her strong sense of Christian duty. I think this must have been inculcated in the years at Lowood, because she never had it before. But Rivers doesn't understand that Jane is also a passionate young girl who needs proper sexual love. Jane can see that he doesn't love her and isn't even physically attracted to her. He wants her to marry him, but only because it wouldn't be respectable for a young woman like her to accompany him only as his 'curate'. Jane refuses this package, although she says she is still willing to go to India as his assistant. We readers breathe a sigh of relief because that won't be allowed. Nevertheless, Rivers continues to work on her with all sorts of moral blackmail. After her refusal he sulks and withholds the brotherly kiss on the cheek that has become a nightly custom. But Jane isn't safe yet. After the loss of Mr Rochester there is a real risk that she might sacrifice herself to this man of stone. Then, just as she seems on the brink of a last-minute surrender, she hears a voice calling 'Jane! Jane! Jane!' It is the voice (in her head) of Rochester and her response is instant: ' "I am coming!" I cried. "Wait for me! Oh, I will come!" ' And the next morning, once again at first light, she makes her escape.

Back at Thornfield Jane is shocked to discover that the Rochester mansion is a burnt-out ruin. She learns from the local innkeeper that there had been a terrible fire in the night several months earlier. No need to ask who started it. As the flames engulfed the house the first Mrs Rochester was seen on the roof, waving and shouting. Mr Rochester tried to reach her but she flung herself over the battlements and was killed. Rochester himself was injured when part of the house collapsed on him. One hand had had to be amputated, he had lost one eye and the other was blind from 'inflammation'. He now resides on an isolated farm 30 miles away.

Happy ending

I will leave you to read and enjoy for yourselves the reunion of our lovers. Jane, of course, isn't in the least bothered by her master's scorched face and sightless eye; she is so happy to be able to care for him. She tidies him up tenderly and combs his hair. She sits on his knee. Did you know a Victorian heroine could do that? When he says, 'Am I hideous, Jane?', she says: 'Very, sir; you always were, you know.' It's so nice to see their old teasing, affectionate relationship restored.

The last chapter begins with the famous line: 'Reader, I married him.' After two years Edward even begins to recover a little of the sight in his remaining eye. With the help of a London oculist he is able to see quite well by the time their first child is born. At this point I always remember that Charlotte Brontë began to write *Jane Eyre* while she was waiting for her father to recover from his cataract extraction.

So Jane's story ends happily, and on the last page Charlotte ties up the loose ends. The Rivers sisters marry happily too and in India St John, still single, toils away at saving souls for Christ. His last letter to Jane indicates that he has not long to live. Jane is comforted by the certainty that he will have his just reward in heaven, as he had always anticipated. This paragraph is written with such apparent fervour that it is hard to know whether Charlotte is being ironic. I think most people fail to notice it as they close the book and sigh contentedly over the picture of Jane sitting on her beloved Mr Rochester's knee, with her arms around his neck.

The text

Jane Eyre by Charlotte Brontë is available in Penguin Classics or Oxford World Classics.

Further reading

- Barker J (1994) *The Brontës.* Phoenix Giants, Weidenfeld and Nicholson, London.

- Gilbert SM and Gubar S (2000) *The Madwoman in the Attic: the woman writer and the nineteenth century literary imagination* (2e). Yale Nota Bene, Yale University Press, New Haven and London.

6

Moby-Dick

by Herman Melville (1851)

This is another of my long-time favourite big books. As I expect you know, it's a tale about a quest for a whale, and you need a big book to deal with such an enormous and awe-inspiring creature. The heart of the book is the story of Captain Ahab and his obsession with the mysterious and terrible white whale which took off his leg in their first encounter; but once you begin you will find that *Moby-Dick* is more than a thrilling sea story. By the time you have finished you will know more about whales and whaling than you ever thought possible; you will also have had an enjoyable time in the company of a brilliant and original writer who seems to know a thing or two about the depths of the human soul as well as those of the Pacific Ocean.

Who was Herman Melville?

Let us start, as we so often do, by getting to know a little about the author. The first thing to say is that he was an American and *Moby-Dick* is probably *the* great American novel. Herman was born in New York City in 1819. His father was a merchant, who unfortunately went bankrupt, lost his reason as well as his money and died when Herman was 12. Mrs Melville had eight children to support altogether, so goodness knows how she managed. The young Herman worked a little at various jobs, went to college a little, couldn't settle down and eventually, at the age of 20, signed on as a merchant seaman for a round trip to Liverpool. After that he tried various other jobs on land (including teaching) before going to sea again, this time on a whaler. He had various adventures, including desertion, mutiny, six months in Honolulu and a year's service with the US Navy, who eventually brought him home. Then he began writing sea stories, which, at first, were very successful. He got married, acquired a country estate and wrote *Moby-Dick* in 1850–51. Unfortunately, his public, who preferred more conventional yarns, didn't take to it. His subsequent novels, *Pierre* and *The Confidence Man*, did not succeed either and, sad to say, his literary career collapsed. After more restless, unhappy years he found a rather melancholy job as a deputy inspector of customs in New York. He continued writing, producing some memorable verse and some excellent short works of fiction, culminating in another sea story, *Billy Budd*, which Benjamin Britten turned into an opera. After his death in 1891 his widow carefully packed the manuscript away and it was not finally discovered and published until 1924.

I realise that my biography makes Herman sound rather miserable, but reading *Moby-Dick* will give you an entirely different impression. This Herman Melville is a lively, exuberant fellow who never stops talking (about whales, the universe and everything) as he grabs us by the hand and tries to haul us off on a desperate and dangerous sea voyage. Shall we join him?

In the library

OK, but hang on a minute. The book begins with two rather eccentric introductions. The first is called 'Etymology' and it consists of three extracts about the origin of the word 'whale', followed by the word for whale in various different languages. This is followed by a visit to the library to see a collection of 'extracts' on the subject of whales and whaling, starting with the Bible and proceeding more or less chronologically through literature and travellers' tales, to reports from whalers themselves in prose and in song. These are quite intriguing, but after a few pages we begin to feel restless. When is the story going to start?

Turn one more page and you reach Chapter 1, which is called 'Loomings'. (Chapter lovers will be pleased to hear that all the chapters have excellent names and most of them are quite short.)

Loomings

Here our storyteller famously introduces himself: 'Call me Ishmael. Some years ago – never mind how long precisely – having little or no money in my purse and nothing particularly to interest me on the shore, I thought I would sail about a little and see the watery part of the world.' This is what he does whenever he gets the 'hypos', which I think here means depressed rather than low on blood glucose. Ishmael tells us he lives in 'the insular city of the Manhattoes' (can you guess where that is?), where all roads lead down to the waterfront and everyone seems to be yearning to go to sea. Then he lets us know that he never sails as a passenger or even an officer but always as a simple sailor 'right before the mast'. He doesn't really mind if they give him a hard time: 'What of it, if some old hunk of a sea-captain orders me to get a broom and sweep the decks? What does that indignity amount to weighed in the scales of the New Testament? Do you think the Archangel Gabriel thinks any less of me …?' Among other reasons for going to sea in this lowly capacity are the fact that he gets paid, and the 'wholesome exercise and pure air of the forecastle deck'. But what persuaded him on this occasion, he asks us, to go for a whaling ship? First, it was a fascination with the whale himself: 'such a portentous and mysterious monster roused all my curiosity. Then the wild and distant sea where he rolled his island bulk; the undeliverable nameless perils of the whale; these with all the attending marvels of a thousand Patagonial sights and sounds, helped to sway me to my wish.' He concludes that 'there floated in my soul endless processions of the whale, and midmost of them all, one grand hooded phantom, like a snow hill in the air'. And with that first hint (or looming) of Moby Dick himself, Ishmael (alias Herman M) concludes this stunning first chapter.

I have shown you quite a large portion of Chapter 1 to give you an idea of what sort of shipmate we have fallen in with here.

I warned you that he talked all the time and some people might find that annoying (I do myself at times). But what a talker he is! His language is grand, rhetorical and argumentative; he beseeches, he preaches, he provokes; he educates you like the schoolmaster he was before he went to sea; he paints you pictures, he sings songs, he cracks jokes, digs you in the ribs, pours icy sea water over you, scares you rigid, fills you with wonder. So what do you say? Is it all a bit much and would you rather go home? Oh come on, let's live dangerously; we'll sling our carpetbags over our shoulders and go with Ishmael.

New Bedford and Nantucket

The whaling business in America was centred on the island of Nantucket, 40 miles off the Massachusetts coast. If you ever get the chance, I recommend a visit to this 'elbow of sand' where you can swim, sail, admire the old sea captains' houses and visit the whaling museum. But we can't go there just yet because Ishmael has missed the boat and has to spend the weekend on the mainland in New Bedford. Here, he puts up at 'The Spouter Inn', where the rooms are all taken and he has to share a bed with a strange, heavily tattooed South Sea Islander called Queequeg. Ishmael, who is not used to meeting people of other nations, is convinced that Queequeg is a cannibal, and he is not reassured by the fact that his roommate has a bag containing a shrunken human head that he has been trying to sell. He also carries a dangerous looking combination tomahawk and pipe, which he likes to smoke in bed. Initially the two men are terrified of each other, but once they have been properly introduced by the landlord, Queequeg calms down and Ishmael realises that this 'savage' is a perfect gentleman. They both sleep soundly and Ishmael wakes to find Queequeg's arm protectively (maybe even a little amorously) embracing him. This strange night at the Spouter Inn enables Ishmael to shed some of his ignorant racial prejudices. He comes to have considerable affection and respect for Queequeg, who turns out to be a very accomplished seaman and harpooneer as well as a thoroughly nice chap once you get to know him.

We sign up for the voyage

Since he has to spend a Sunday in New Bedford, Ishmael goes to chapel and listens to a magnificent sermon (the text, you will not be surprised to hear, is from the book of Jonah). During the day he and Queequeg do a bit more bonding and on Monday morning the two friends catch the packet boat for Nantucket. Here they put up at another inn, The Trypots, well known for the quality of its chowder. There is a choice of clam or cod – and you would be foolish not to take the opportunity of sampling them both. On the next day, they go about the important task of choosing a whaling ship on which to enlist. Queequeg says that his little black god Yojo (yet another of his intriguing personal possessions) has told him that Ishmael should go first to the docks, where he will be infallibly guided to the right ship. Ishmael is not entirely convinced but off he goes and picks out the *Pequod*. She is rather a grotesque, battle-scarred-looking ship, but Ishmael is rather taken with her. On board the ship he finds two old salts, Captain Peleg and Captain Bildad, who are part owners of the *Pequod*. Peleg subjects Ishmael to an interrogation about his sea-going experience and finally signs him on at the very low rate of 'the 275th lay', which means one two hundred and seventy-fifth part of the net profits of the voyage, this being the way in which whaling ships paid their crews. When Queequeg saunters down, later in the day, he impresses the two old captains by accurately impaling, with a throw of his harpoon, a small patch of tar floating on the water; as a much more valuable member of the team he is immediately offered the 90th lay. A whaler would have a crew of about 30 men altogether. I will leave you to do the maths.

Ishmael also learns that when the *Pequod* sets sail she will be commanded by the legendary Captain Ahab, who has lately been 'a kind of moody' since his loss of a leg in an attempt to catch the notorious white whale called Moby Dick. Not just moody, but 'desperate moody, and savage sometimes'. However, Ishmael is assured by Captain Peleg that it is 'better to sail with a moody good captain than a laughing bad one'. And so, in Chapter 22, at Christmas, perhaps even on Christmas Day, the *Pequod* set sail, left its pilot boat behind at the harbour mouth and 'blindly plunged like fate into the lone Atlantic'. We are off!

Meet Captain Ahab and the crew of the *Pequod*

As we are sailing along, Ishmael (or is it Melville), in a chapter called 'The advocate', puts the case for whaling being a worthy subject for a writer. The whale is 'a royal fish' and whaling was, at the time, still an important industry. Nowadays, we are more than happy to watch whales, but want to see them protected and preserved rather than brutally murdered, dismembered and melted down. On this voyage we are all looking forward to seeing the whales, but some of us (and I include myself here) are rather squeamish about what Captain Ahab and his crew are going to do to them. We shall, of course, return to this problem. But now it's time to meet the *Pequod*'s officers. There are three mates, called Starbuck, Stubb and Flask, all with very different personalities. Starbuck, the senior, is calm and steadfast; courageous but cautious. He doesn't believe that lives should be unnecessarily put at risk for a single whale while there are plenty more in the sea. Stubb, the second mate, is a happy-go-lucky fellow who sings to himself and likes to make himself comfortable. He smokes a small black pipe, which he keeps going even while chasing a whale in a small boat. The third mate, Flask, is 'a short, stout, ruddy young fellow, very pugnacious concerning whales'. Now this is the way the whale hunting works. Each of the three mates is the commander of a small boat, which is lowered as soon as a whale is sighted. When the boats set out the mate is steering and everyone else is rowing. Each mate has his regular harpooneer or boat-steerer, whose job is to stand precariously in the front of the boat and hurl the harpoon (a long spear attached to a line), which will catch in the whale's side like a great fish hook and prevent him escaping. He then changes places with the mate and becomes the boat-steerer while the mate takes command of the capturing and killing of the unfortunate whale. You will note that all the harpooneers are non-white Americans: Queequeg (whom we know already), Tashtego (an American Indian) and Daggoo, a giant African American who wears large gold earrings like ring bolts. Ishmael introduces us to all these interesting people; meanwhile, on the quarter deck we may catch sight of Captain Ahab, his peg leg (carved from a whale's jaw bone) firmly wedged in a special socket in the planking, his bearing erect and his eye 'looking straight out beyond the ship's ever-pitching prow'.

A lecture on whales and their classification

In Chapter 32 (called 'Cetology'), Ishmael begins a series of lectures on the whale. I do recommend you to take this course, which is an important part of your education, covering the anatomy, physiology, psychology, natural history and industrial application of the whale. Now a modern-day cetologist would certainly find fault with Ishmael's classification, but the main thing to grasp is the difference between the sperm whale and the right (or whalebone) whale. The right whale is the one with a kind of cartilaginous Venetian blind construction in its mouth, with which it filters out the nutritious plankton from seawater. The sperm whale, on the other hand, has proper teeth and a large, domed head, whose upper part contains a large tank full of a very fine oil called spermaceti, which the Victorians used to make special candles and perfume. A sperm whale is about 60 feet long and the size of two double-decker buses.

Ahab is obsessed with Moby Dick

A few leagues further on, Ahab calls all the ship's company aft and addresses them. He nails a gold doubloon (worth 16 dollars) to the main-mast and tells them that the first man to spot Moby Dick will be able to claim the coin as a reward. It becomes clear that he is only interested in one whale now and that is Moby Dick; it's not business, it's personal. But how about the rest of us, who thought this was a routine whaling trip? '"And this is what ye shipped for, men!" (cries the captain) "to chase that white whale on both sides of land, and over all sides of earth, till he spits black blood and rolls fin out. What say, men, will ye splice hands on it, now? I think ye do look brave." '

Sensible Mr Starbuck is appalled. '"Vengeance on a dumb brute!" cried Starbuck, "that simply smote thee from blindest instinct! Madness!" ' But there is no talking to Captain Ahab. His heart is filled with hatred for his enemy. Just who is Captain Ahab? The depth and violence of his passions suggest a more than human, demonic 'hero', a sort of sea-going Heathcliff (who is his near contemporary in literature).

Ahab now conducts a weird ceremony in which the three mates offer grog to the three harpooneers using the sockets of their harpoons as cups. ' "Death to Moby Dick" ' shouts the entire crew: 'The long barbed steel goblets were lifted and to cries and maledictions against the white whale, the spirits were simultaneously quaffed down with a hiss.'

I had a feeling we should not have boarded this ship in the first place: it's a bit too much like the one in *The Rime of the Ancient Mariner* for comfort. But it's too late now.

The captain and the whale

The ship sails on. Melville records the passage of the next night in soliloquy (Starbuck), songs and a dramatisation (the entire company). Then we come to an important chapter (Chapter 41) entitled simply 'Moby Dick'. Ishmael fills us in on some of the legends surrounding the monster. He is not only large and distinctive; he is known to be ferocious, cunning and spiteful. Every attempt to catch him so far has come to grief: boats stove in and sunk, terrible injuries, loss of human life. There is also something of the supernatural about him. Sailors say that he is immortal and ubiquitous: if he is killed in one ocean he will only surface again in another part of the globe. How can you identify him if you see him? He is not only very large, he has a crooked jaw, 'a peculiar snow-white wrinkled forehead and a high, pyramidical white hump'. And his body is bristling with the twisted remains of the harpoons with which numerous whalers have tried in vain to kill him. Melville goes on to tell us in an unforgettable three and a half pages of spine-tingling writing just how terrible is the hatred of the whale with which Ahab is consumed: 'He piled upon the whale's white hump the sum of all the general hate and rage felt by his whole race from Adam down; and then, as if his chest had been a mortar, he burst his hot heart's shell upon it.' That's just a sample; you absolutely have to experience all the wonderful phrases Melville uses to describe our poor crazed captain's condition: 'Gnawed within and scorched without, with the infixed fangs of some incurable idea.'

'The whiteness of the whale'

Then the mood changes. In another award-winning chapter, Herman Melville broods on the qualities of whiteness – why is it so terrifying? He offers numerous examples for us to consider. Think of 'sailing through a midnight sea of milky whiteness' (with rocks lurking beneath); or the frosty whiteness of remote high mountains; or the snowy wastes of the prairie in winter. Or, worst of all, imagine the ghastly whiteness of a world totally without colour. The huge, white whale now seems to represent the pitiless vastness of the universe. Chapter 45 finds us in Captain Ahab's cabin, looking over his shoulder as he plots the likely course and position of his enemy – taking into account the ocean currents and tides, the whale feeding grounds and what he knows about Moby Dick's preferred cruising patterns. Is it possible to find a single whale in all the oceans of the world? Ahab seems to think so. First of all, Moby Dick is easy to recognise, and there have been documented accounts of his having deliberately attacked other whaling ships. These encounters have mostly occurred during Moby Dick's favourite 'season-on-the-line', a time of year he likes to spend in the equatorial regions of the Pacific. To convince us of the hostile intentions of certain sperm whales he quotes the true story of the whale ship *Essex*, which was attacked by a furious whale who 'dashed his forehead' against the ship and sank her in 10 minutes. The story of the *Essex*, well known to all whale men, may have given Melville the inspiration for *Moby-Dick*. You can read about the fate of the crew of the *Essex* in a book called *In the Heart of the Sea* by Nathaniel Philbrick, published in 2000.

I will just pause to note that today's whale lovers (and again I include myself) might well think the animal in question was acting in very justifiable self-defence, considering that the *Essex*'s crew had already killed several of his family and friends and were intent on doing the same to him. But in those days, the men's livelihood depended on hunting the whales and selling their oil: the whales were expected to understand this and to accept their fate gracefully.

There she blows!

Now the whale-chasing and killing is about to begin, so I must warn those of you who are feeling squeamish as well as seasick to swallow a couple of stemetils and try to be brave. From his look-out post at the masthead, Tashtego, the harpooneer, cries 'There she blows!' The first whale has been sighted and the boats are lowered. One boat is commanded by each mate, but to everyone's surprise the captain has secretly taken on an additional harpooneer and crew for a boat of his own. The first chase is very exciting. We are in Starbuck's boat with Queequeg as harpooneer. You should realise that these boats are only 30 feet long, while an adult sperm whale could be 60–80 feet from his brow to his flukes. There is a squall approaching as we get near the whales, Queequeg's harpoon fails to lodge and the boat is swamped by the squall. The *Pequod* looms up through the mist and everyone dives into the water in terror just before the big ship crushes the little boat. But we all get hauled back safely onto the mother ship. We are freezing cold and saturated with sea-water and some of us have post traumatic stress disorder but we are OK. What's next?

The killing of a whale

In the next few chapters we sail round the Cape of Good Hope and have a mid-ocean meeting with another whaler (*The Town-Ho*). We hear a thrilling and chilling tale of a leaking ship, a grievance, a mutiny cruelly suppressed and the thirst for vengeance, all culminating in an encounter with Moby Dick in a mean mood! This tale within a tale I must leave you to read for yourselves, because it's time for us to continue our apprenticeship in whaling. More whales are sighted and this time we are in Mr Stubb's boat. His harpooneer successfully lodges his weapon in a sperm whale's body and the animal is held fast by the long line which whips out of the boat as the whale tries to escape. The whale is at last hauled close to the boat (or the boat to the whale) and Stubb proceeds to stab it repeatedly with his long lance. This is horrible, especially for herbivores. The water bubbles and boils with blood. Finally the huge animal is stabbed in the heart, blood gushes out of its spout-hole and it is dead. It's a brilliant and thrilling description, so you have to read it even as you mourn the sad death of the noble and innocent creature.

Cutting in

The next part of the business we have to learn is how the whalers get the valuable parts of their victim on board the ship in a manageable form. The whale's skin, as you know, has a massive layer of oily subcutaneous fat, which can be melted down to yield barrels of oil. The dead whale is tied to the side of the ship and someone has to stand precariously on its back and stick in a huge hook. The hook is attached to a line and when a flap of blubber-laden skin around the hook has been dissected free, a huge piece is stripped off and hauled up on to the ship by a winch. The ship keels over alarmingly with the weight of the whale as the heavy strip of blubber is torn off and pulled on board. The process goes on until all that is left is a skinned carcase. Then the whale is decapitated and the body cast adrift for the sharks. The head of a sperm whale must be kept because it contains the most valuable prize of all: the chamber full of precious aromatic spermaceti oil. This mysterious substance can only be obtained by climbing inside the head and baling the oil out with a bucket on the end of a rope. All this will be described by Ishmael in vivid detail. Later on you will also witness the bizarre scenes of 'trying out', in which the strips of blubber are cut into manageable chunks and melted down in huge iron 'try pots' heated on wood-fuelled fires (red flames; thick, choking black smoke; hideous smells) before finally being decanted into wooden barrels to take home for sale in Nantucket.

The anatomy lesson

At one point (Chapter 74) the *Pequod* has a sperm whale's head suspended from one side and a right whale's head hung on the other. Now the *Pequod*'s crew normally scorn the right whale and don't bother with it. But it is said that a ship which has hung a head of each kind on either side will never be capsized, so it's worth catching at least one. While they are both hanging there, Ishmael the anatomy professor takes the opportunity of conducting us round both heads, pointing out the important differences. Our cetology curriculum continues in the intervals between further whale hunts (for the business must go on if we are to make any money out of this trip). There is a chapter on the fountain: did you know that the right whale has two spout holes, while the sperm whale has only one? And what exactly comes out of those huge nostrils? Is it breath alone or air and water? There's another great lecture on the tail and the things a whale can do with those muscular horizontal flukes. Don't miss it. There is even a chapter devoted to the whale's foreskin. (I kid you not, it's Chapter 95 and it's called 'The Cassock', for reasons which will become clear when you read it.)

If you prefer to study your whales while they are alive, and see a glimpse of their domestic life, you will enjoy Chapter 87 ('The Grand Armada'), in which one of the boats is pulled into the middle of a huge 'armada' of sperm whales all travelling together. Here in the centre, everything is calm and the juvenile whales play innocently around the killer boat, coming up to have their heads scratched by Queequeg. In the depths, the men can just make out the mother whales suckling their young, who look up at the men, just like human babies, while continuing to feed. This remarkable chapter provides a peaceful and moving contrast to the scenes of bloody carnage which surround it. You have the impression that even the hardened whaling men might be wondering why they should have to spend their lives attacking and slaughtering these beautiful, almost mythic creatures.

The castaway

While we are in this part of the book, I must mention the story of little Pip (Chapter 93, 'The Castaway'). Pip is a little black boy who jumps out of a boat in terror just as the whale is harpooned. He gets tangled up in the line and Stubb, after some hesitation, orders him to be cut free 'so that the whale was lost and Pip was free'. Stubb warns him that if he jumps again he won't be saved because a whale is worth 30 times as much as he is. 'But we are all in the hands of the Gods; and Pip jumped again.' In the end he is saved, but only after a terrifying period of lonesome swimming in the awful emptiness of the Pacific a mile from the ship. After that, sad to say, he is never quite right in the head. The ocean has shown him things that no human being can bear.

Towards the end of the voyage

The *Pequod* sails on. More whales are chased and caught. But as far as Ahab is concerned there is only one whale that matters. He gets the ship's carpenter to make him a new peg leg and the black-smith to forge him a new harpoon. In an encounter with another ship he meets an English captain who has lost an arm in a struggle with Moby Dick – and sports a whale-ivory replacement, which complements Ahab's prosthetic leg. The two traumatised captains clash their ivory limbs together in a ghastly greeting. This rather humorous chapter also introduces the English captain's surgeon (at last a doctor hoves in sight! I thought one was never coming). The English captain is full of praise for Dr Bunger's treatment: 'I'd rather be killed by you than kept alive by any other man.'

After a variety of other diversions and tutorials (whale skeletons, fossil whales, will the whale perish?) the *Pequod* passes through the China Sea and into the Pacific proper. We are almost in the Japanese Cruising Ground where Ahab expects to find Moby Dick at last. But before that happens the crew have to endure a night-marish thunderstorm in which balls of lightning ('corpusants') are seen at the yardarms and 'each of the tall three masts was silently burning in that sulphurous air like three gigantic wax tapers before an altar'. Again, it's all getting horribly like *The Rime of the Ancient Mariner.* Finally, Ahab's harpoon fixed in the prow of his whaling boat starts to shoot out 'a levelled flame of pale forked fire'. The crew are terrified but Ahab calmly seizes the harpoon and blows out the fire with his mighty breath.

Will Ahab give it up and go home? Can Starbuck persuade him?

Now we are getting very near to the end of the book and Ahab's final settlement with the White Whale. In Chapter 128, the *Pequod* meets the *Rachel,* whose captain confirms that they have sighted and chased Moby Dick and may even have stuck a harpoon in him – although he got away. But sad to say, one of their boats is missing and it contained the captain's young son. His father begs Ahab to let him charter the *Pequod* for 48 hours so that the two ships can search for him – but Ahab refuses. He can't bear the thought of losing Moby Dick even for the sake of a fellow captain's child. Curiously, at this point he adopts a 'son' of his own: little Pip takes up residence in the captain's cabin, where Ahab insists that he stays, although Pip wants to follow him up on deck.

In Chapter 122 ('The Symphony'), it's a beautiful day with a clear blue sky and Ahab experiences a little window of sanity. We dare to hope that he might realise the madness of his mission and give it up. In a heart-stopping monologue he pours out his feelings to Starbuck, the first mate; Ahab tells him he has been whaling for 40 years and during all that time he has not spent three years ashore. He reflects on the young wife he has left behind 'leaving but one dent in my marriage pillow'. She is like a widow with a husband alive. The old man is close to tears as he admits 'what a forty years fool' he has been.

Starbuck's heart floods with sudden hope: ' "Oh my Captain! my Captain! noble soul! Grand old heart, after all! Why should anyone give chase to that hated fish! Away with me! Let us fly these deadly waters! Let us home!" ' It's moving. It's gripping. But it's no good. Ahab soon reverts to his usual mad, driven self and the chase is on.

The final showdown

That night, Ahab sniffs something in the wind and he just knows that a big sperm whale is near. He orders a change of course and soon Moby Dick himself is sighted from all three mast-heads. The chase is on and it will occupy three thrilling chapters until the final outcome is known. And at this point, dear readers, I am going to leave you. I have secretly ordered a ship of my own to rendezvous with us here and take me back to Nantucket. I shall leave you to discover for yourselves what happens in the final showdown between the crazed old seadog and the wicked old whale. Stay with Ishmael – he will look after you. Have a wonderful time and don't forget to wear your lifejackets.

Below the waterline: deeper meanings in *Moby-Dick*

I have already hinted that Melville's masterpiece is more than a thrilling sea-story and an encyclopaedia of whaling. And you will have noticed that Ishmael's thoughts and speculations often widen to address the big questions like how we poor humans manage to make sense of our lives as we float like mere specks of krill on the surface of our watery planet. Ever since it was written, scholars have been puzzling over the 'true' meaning of *Moby-Dick*. Some have seen it as the story of the exploration of America with the pioneers, like Ahab, determined to conquer the huge and dangerous continent. Alternatively, you can see Captain Ahab as a deranged dictator whose ways of relating are contrasted with those of the forecastle, where a spirit of democracy and equality unites the crew. You will have noticed that while Ishmael at first finds the non-white sailors strange, he soon begins to treat them simply as fellow human beings. Everyone is valued and there is really no racism on board the *Pequod*. It's just like the American ideal of the melting pot where everyone becomes a citizen. Is this Melville's way of reacting to the tensions in America about racial inequality, which would result in the Civil War? Or should we take a more psychodynamic view and see the White Whale as a massive projection of all the anger and destructiveness which lurk in the human unconscious and which we would like to have personified and demonised in a form which we can easily fear, hate and attack. Is Moby Dick the ultimate terrorist against whom President Ahab is waging war? I shall stretch the comparison no further. Whatever your thoughts about the deeper meanings of *Moby-Dick*, the most important thing is that it is a whale of a book, there for you to read and to enjoy.

The text

Moby-Dick or, The Whale by Herman Melville is available in the Penguin Classics edition with an introduction by Andrew Delbanco and excellent notes by Tom Quirk.

7

Fathers and Sons

by Ivan Turgenev (1862)

Everyone has heard of Tolstoy and Dostoyevsky, the great shaggy bears of nineteenth-century Russian literature; but their contemporary Ivan Turgenev is not so well known to today's English readers. And yet, his novel *Fathers and Sons,* when it was published in 1862, caused a greater storm of controversy than any other Russian novel before or since. Just why this happened, we will shortly discover. And if you haven't yet read *Fathers and Sons*, I shall have the pleasure of introducing you to a moving, memorable and perfectly written story, which you will at once award an honoured place on your shelves alongside *Anna Karenina* and *The Brothers Karamazov.*

A biographical sketch

Ivan Turgenev was born in 1818, the son of a retired cavalry officer and a rich heiress. He spent his childhood on their large country estate, where he witnessed the extreme harshness and cruelty with which his mother treated the peasants. This experience left him with a deep and enduring dislike of injustice and tyranny. After studying at the universities of Moscow and St Petersburg, he went to Berlin to learn philosophy. He met a number of other young Russian intellectuals who were becoming fired up by revolutionary political ideas. He also developed a great devotion to Western culture.

Back in Russia, Turgenev became a writer, but remained very concerned about the need for social and political change in Russia. He knew all the fiery young radicals of the day but he especially admired the political writer and literary critic Vissarion Belinsky. Belinsky was passionate about literature, but he also believed that writers should be politically committed and that literature had to be an agent of moral and social reform. Turgenev himself had a different view of literature, as we shall shortly see. His first book, *The Sportsman's Sketches* (1852), was a loosely linked collection of stories in which he portrayed the subjugated Russian peasants as more humane and sensitive than their masters. This got him into deep trouble with the authorities. It was even thought to have influenced the new Tsar Alexander III to order the emancipation (freeing) of all the serfs in 1861. Further novels followed, and also a play called *A Month in the Country*, which is still performed regularly.

Turgenev's literary career prospered. The liberals were pleased by his commitment to social justice and the conservatives admired his elegant writing and lively characterisation. Turgenev seemed to be liked by everybody. Unfortunately, *Fathers and Sons* upset readers on both sides because of the character Bazarov, who seemed to be a portrait of a typical Russian socialist, forthright, ruthless and arrogant, but possibly speaking the truth, depending on your politics. Dismayed by the sustained abuse that was suddenly being hurled at him, Turgenev retreated to Europe, where he spent most of the rest of his life until 1880. In France, Germany and England he received much kinder treatment. Flaubert and Henry James both admired him, and Oxford University gave him an honorary doctorate in 1879. He was a tall, elegant fellow, who was always exquisitely dressed and enjoyed all the good things of life. He had a lifelong passion for a beautiful Spanish opera singer called Pauline Viardot and pursued her all over Europe. She was already married, but her husband seemed not to mind. After a long illness, Turgenev died in Paris in 1893. At his request, he was buried in St Petersburg near his old friend and mentor, Belinsky.

Fathers and Sons: the homecoming

Now let's have a look at the book that caused poor Turgenev so much grief. The first person we meet is 'a gentleman of just over forty years of age, in a dusty overcoat and check trousers'. This is Nicholas Kirsanov, who is waiting with his manservant at a roadside inn for the arrival of his beloved son, Arcady. Nicholas is in a state of great excitement because Arcady has just finished his three years at the University of St Petersburg and is coming home to begin a new life as a graduate. Those of us over 50 are a little disconcerted to find that Arcady's forty-ish father is described as 'a grizzled, slightly bent, stoutish elderly gentleman'. While we are waiting for the coach to arrive, Turgenev gives a lightning sketch of Nicholas's life so far: he was the son of wealthy landowners and he had followed his father into a military career, but soon gave it up. He had married for love and he and his wife had enjoyed a happy life playing duets on the piano, planting flowers and keeping chickens. Sadly his wife died after ten years, leaving Nicholas with Arcady, their only child. And look, here he comes now: a young man is jumping out of a *tarantass* (a small, four-wheeled carriage pulled by three horses) and warmly embracing his dad. But there is another young man with him: Arcady has brought home a friend.

A friend from college

The friend introduces himself as Eugene Vasilich Bazarov; he has a long, gaunt face with a broad forehead, greenish eyes and bushy whiskers. He has a serene smile and seems both intelligent and self-assured. We can't help noticing that he is also rather brusque and lacking in social graces.

Arcady tells his father that Bazarov is a natural scientist who is about to take his medical degree. So he's a medical student! We want to hear more, but we must wait a little. As they ride along, Arcady can't help noticing that the estate is rather run down and neglected-looking. His father confides that he is having a lot of trouble with the newly liberated serfs, who won't pay their rent.

Arcady also learns that a certain young servant girl with whom his father has been having an affair has now been brought into the house to live with him. Nicholas is acutely embarrassed at having to make this revelation, but his son is not in the least bothered. Why shouldn't the old man live with his girlfriend? No problem for the younger generation. When they arrive at the house, Arcady is greeted by Paul, his father's elder brother. Uncle Paul is about 44, dapper, beautifully dressed and with perfect manners. A bit like Turgenev himself, perhaps. He catches sight of Bazarov and is not favourably impressed by the young man's uncouth appearance. 'Is he staying with us?' he asks. 'That hairy creature?' As for Bazarov, he regards the elegant, middle-aged gentleman as a huge joke. But Arcady is ever so pleased to be home again and he and his friend are soon peacefully asleep. The two older men remain awake for longer, Nicholas excited about his son's return, Paul feeling unsettled by the arrival of the hairy one. At the end of his description of the house settling down for the night, Turgenev gives us a wonderful little cameo, like a Dutch painting, of Nicholas's young mistress, Fenichka, dressed in a warm, pale blue knitted jumper and white kerchief, sitting and listening to the breathing of her baby.

What do you mean, you're a nihilist?

In the morning, Bazarov rises early, has a quick tour of the gardens and stables and then goes off to a nearby marsh, accompanied by two servants whom he has recruited to help him to catch frogs. 'What's the frogs for, master?' asks one of the peasants. And Bazarov says: 'I'll split a frog open and see what's going on inside. Except for the fact that we walk about on our hind legs, we are very like these frogs and that will help me to learn what is going on inside us too.'

He describes himself as a doctor so I guess we will have to accept him as one of us, even though he is not yet fully qualified. You will have noticed from his intentions towards the frogs that he believes in empirical research rather than traditional beliefs. Is he an early advocate of evidence-based medicine? I think he probably is, and with attitude to match, as we shall shortly see.

Meanwhile, back at the house, Arcady tells his father that there is no need to be ashamed of his love for Fenichka. He goes to find her and makes friends with her and the baby, whom he is very happy to welcome as his little brother. Now, Uncle Paul comes down to breakfast in his English morning coat and his smoking-cap. He quizzes Arcady about his medical student friend and Arcady tells him that Bazarov is 'a Nihilist', a term actually launched by Turgenev himself to describe the 1860s generation of intellectuals. The two old gentlemen (I know they are only in their forties but they behave like old gentlemen) are aghast. A nihilist? A man who believes in nothing? That's terrible! But Arcady says it means someone who 'looks at everything critically'. A nihilist is 'a man who admits no established authorities, who takes no principles for granted, however much they may be respected'. The brothers are not persuaded that such an attitude is a Good Thing. Relations become even more strained when Bazarov tells them that 'a good chemist is more useful than a score of poets'. On the other hand, he doesn't believe in science 'in general' either. Uncle Paul tries to pursue the matter of what Bazarov does and does not believe in even further, but the uncouth young man snaps back: 'What is this, a cross-examination?' Nicholas intervenes and the two old boys retreat, Paul muttering as if to himself, 'One does one's best to remember what one has been taught, but it all turns out to be rubbish.' It reminds me very much of the first arrival on our medical scene of the nihilists of evidence-based medicine. I mean we've always given children antibiotics for earache and it seems to work. How can they suddenly say: 'you should stop because there's no evidence'?

Getting to know the family

In the next chapter (Chapter 7), Arcady tells Bazarov his uncle's rather melancholy history. He relates how Paul, as a young officer, fell heavily in love with a married society woman who finally rejected him. After ten years of pursuit he finally admitted defeat, but by then his life had lost its momentum. He just settled down in his brother's house to a bachelor life of good books, fine wines, nice clothes and perfect manners. All the local ladies think he is a very romantic old gentleman. He sounds a bit like the author himself, but with the big difference that Turgenev was also a great writer. Bazarov is not in the least touched by Uncle Paul's romantic history and says he would rather go off and examine an interesting beetle.

Next, we hear about how Arcady's father (Nicholas) met and fell in love with Fenichka. Bazarov also gets acquainted with Fenichka and, in his medical capacity, checks out baby Mitya's teething problems. Although she is usually very shy with the gentry, Fenichka finds Bazarov very easy to get on with; and he is really kind and helpful. We begin to feel that he is not such a bad chap after all. He even tells Arcady that he approves his father's action in bringing his little peasant family into the house – although, as we would expect, he attaches no importance to the institution of marriage. Then he rather spoils the good impression he is making by laughing at Nicholas for playing the cello at the age of forty-odd. I think it's the romantic melancholy that presumably goes with solitary cello-playing in the country that Bazarov finds absurd – but Arcady is rather hurt to hear his father ridiculed by his friend and mentor.

Life in Marino: a clash of values

After a while, life in Marino seems to centre on Bazarov. The student nihilist works away at chemistry and gazes down his microscope, with periodic excursions to gather herbs and insects. Nicholas finds him rather frightening and worries about his influence on his son, but is willing to help him with his experiments. Fenichka likes him and so do the servants. Only Uncle Paul has developed a violent dislike for Bazarov (whose first name, by the way, is Eugene). But Eugene continues to be abrasive. He tells Arcady that his father is a good-natured old boy but a complete has-been. '"A couple of days ago I caught him reading Pushkin", Bazarov went on meanwhile. "Will you please explain to him that this won't do? He's no youth, it's time he gave up such nonsense."' Now Pushkin is the nationally revered father of Russian literature, so for anyone with a love for poetry this sort of attitude amounts to blasphemy. To make matters worse, the arrogant boy carries off Pushkin and leaves poor Nicholas with a copy of *Stoff und Kraft*, a work by Ludwig Büchner, which was the key text for the 1860s Russian materialists.

Then Uncle Paul and Nicholas get into a terrible argument with the boys (well, mainly Bazarov) about the aristocracy. Paul sees the aristocrats (among whom he counts himself) as noble fellows who know their rights but fulfil their obligations. 'I may live in the country', says Paul but 'I respect the man in myself'. Eugene points out rather rudely that since Paul just sits in the country 'doing nothing' it really makes no difference to anyone whether he respects himself or not. Paul turns pale at the insult, but Bazarov is just getting started. He is soon telling the two old has-beens that he has no time for words like 'aristocracy, liberalism, progress or principles'. Oh yes, and the Arts can be junked at the same time. The older men are appalled; surely he must be in favour of something. What will he put in the place of the old values? But Bazarov says that he and his friends are not concerned with construction: 'that is not our affair .... First, we must make a clean sweep.'

This was the policy of the revolutionary Russian thinkers such as Belinsky and Bakunin, with whom Turgenev was friendly. But when they read *Fathers and Sons* and found themselves represented by Bazarov, they suspected that their views were being sent up. And the conservatives, who regarded Turgenev as a member of their class who had gone to the bad, were equally sure that he was pouring scorn on the older generation and advocating nihilism. When they challenged him to say which side he was really on, poor Turgenev insisted that he had written a novel, not a manifesto, and that he was on everyone's side. And so he is: his warm empathy for all his characters is partly what makes him such a wonderful storyteller.

The trouble with young people today

As we read about the fierce argument, we begin to appreciate how deeply wounded the older men, especially Paul, feel when confronted with these shocking ideas about what is supposed to be good for 'The Russian People'. As Paul tries and fails to get Bazarov to admit to believing in anything or anybody, the argument gets more heated and, I'm sorry to say, more personal. Finally, the young men withdraw and the two brothers are left to reflect sadly on 'young people today'. Nicholas has enough insight to remember how he once accused his own mother of being unable to understand the younger generation. But Paul doesn't see it and remains in a bad temper.

The next chapter is a lovely one and very much calmer. In it we follow Nicholas's stream of consciousness as he strolls in the garden and reflects on the divide between fathers and sons. Surely what they say can't be right, he thinks; but they seem to have some advantage over us. Is it just that they are so young? No, it can't be that. Perhaps they have fewer traces of the serf master in their character. ' "But to reject poetry?" he asked himself again. "To lack all feeling for art, for nature …".' I do see what he means. Then he falls into a reverie and thinks sadly about his wife, who died so young. He hears Fenichka's voice calling him and he remembers how old he is compared to her. He is overcome with a romantic sadness; which his sharper, sterner brother does not share.

Two young men in search of adventure

Now the two young men decide to take off for a while by themselves as Arcady's home and family are getting a bit boring: 'The young folks at Marino regretted their departure … but the older men breathed a sigh of relief.' In the nearby town they meet various people whom they find rather tedious, including a minister from St Petersburg (who knows Arcady's father) and an embarrassingly stupid disciple of Bazarov. They visit the house of an aristocratic lady with 'progressive' views, who professes an interest in chemistry. But Bazarov is chiefly interested in drinking her Champagne. 'Are there any attractive women in this town?' he asks as he drains his third glass.

A few days later they go to a ball and meet an attractive woman. Her name is Anna Odintzov; she is 29 (older than our young men) and a widow. She is not only beautiful, she is educated and able to think for herself. Something about Turgenev's description of her – I think it's the black dress and the glossy bare arms and the 'barely perceptible smile' – reminds me of Anna Karenina. Arcady dances with her and tells her about his friend. Anna says she is 'very curious to meet a man who dares to believe in nothing'. Bazarov finds her cold and reserved, and he thinks that 'free-thinking women are monstrosities', but he admits to being very taken with her beautiful white shoulders. The next day the two friends call on Anna at her magnificent home. Her husband has left her very well provided for and she enjoys wrapping herself in luxury and comfort. Turgenev, as usual, gives us a little sketch of Anna's history to go with the others in our portfolio. She and Bazarov discuss medicine, homeopathy and botany, and Anna invites them both to come and visit at her country estate. Both young men are quite strongly attracted to her, although Bazarov maintains he is interested only in her body, which he says is 'just ripe for the dissecting table'. This is too much for Arcady, who tells him to shut up. We notice that Arcady is gradually finding less to admire and more to worry about in his friend's personality.

A fortnight at Nicolskoye

They drive over to Nicolskoye (Anna's country house) the next day. In the lavishly furnished house they also meet Anna's formidable old aunt, the Princess K, and her younger sister, Katya. Anna tells Bazarov, 'You had better come closer, and then we can start an argument about something.' (It's a bit like the sketch in *Monty Python* where people pay to have an argument with John Cleese.) So they start an argument about why Bazarov has no use for art. Anna says that an artistic sense might help him to read people's characters. But Bazarov maintains that all human beings are made the same way (like trees). And why would you want to tell one from another? Besides, after the revolution, 'in a properly functioning society, it won't matter whether people are stupid or intelligent, good or bad'.

Meanwhile Arcady has been left out of this high-powered discussion; Anna remembers him and asks her little sister, Katya, to play something for him on the piano. Katya plays him Mozart's Sonata Fantasia in C minor, and not too badly. Whenever a piece of music is mentioned in a novel I run to my CD collection and try to find the piece in question so I know what they are listening to. I recommend that you do the same. All Mozart's piano sonatas are sublime, but critics agree that this fantasia is rather special with its foreshadowing of Beethoven. No wonder Arcady begins to fall just a little bit in love.

That night, Anna reclines in her sumptuous bed, on lace pillows, beneath a silk quilt, thinking about Bazarov. 'What an odd doctor!' she says to herself. And she smiles, reads a little and then falls asleep, as Turgenev says, 'all pure and frigid in her spotless and fragrant linen'. Will Bazarov try to conquer this self-sufficient princess? Unusually for him, he gets quite excited. He can't stop thinking about Anna and what it would be like to make love to her. Arcady thinks he is in love with her too and is madly jealous of the way Anna and Bazarov are always together. In fact, he spends most of his time with sister Katya who is much nicer and easier to get on with.

Anna and Bazarov continue to flirt dangerously with each other. He wants to know 'why does a woman of your intelligence and your beauty live in the country?' And she wants to know how a man like him can really expect to be satisfied with the life of a country doctor. As usual Bazarov gives nothing away. When he finally makes a passionate declaration of love to Anna and tries to embrace her, she half responds and then suddenly rejects him, saying, 'You misunderstood me.' His expression, she thought as he rushed towards her, had been 'almost bestial'. ' "No," she resolved at last, "God knows where that might have led, it's no joking matter. A quiet life is better than anything else in the world." ' I think this is very sad, and I am afraid that this rejection will mark the beginning of a downward path for Bazarov.

Now meet Bazarov's parents

Eugene is furious with himself for having given way to the kind of romantic impulses he usually despises. He decides to leave Nicolskoye at once and pay an overdue visit to his parents. Eugene's father is delighted to see his son again and his mother is practically fainting with joy. Well, it is three years since they have seen their baby. These two seem to be in their sixties, and thus of an older generation than Arcady's father and uncle. Eugene's father is a retired army doctor with many tales to tell of distinguished patients. His mother is 'a genuine Russian gentle-woman of the old school'. She is very devout and superstitious, but also kind-hearted and an excellent cook. Of course she worships her little boy and is all over him. Bazarov, to his credit, is very kind and gentle with her, allowing her to kiss and embrace him without getting too irritable. 'In our time,' Turgenev notes, 'women like her have grown rare. God alone knows whether this is a matter for rejoicing.'

Arcady quite enjoys himself at the Bazarovs. He tells the old man, 'Your son is one of the most remarkable men I have ever met.' They agree that Eugene hates any kind of expression of the emotions, but all the same he is thoroughly honest and unselfish and is destined for great things. Nevertheless, when the two friends get together later in the day, Arcady becomes quite disturbed by Bazarov's dark state of mind and his increasingly extreme statements. In fact, we can see that he is still feeling very wounded by Anna's rejection of his love, although it's hard for him to admit to having such feelings. Instead he goes on about the need to be 'a real man' who must be 'either obeyed or hated'. Poor Bazarov is beginning to hate everyone, even the peasants with their legitimate aspirations for self-improvement. When he calls Arcady's Uncle Paul 'an idiot', Arcady is really angry with him and the two boys nearly come to blows. Fortunately they are interrupted by the genial arrival of Eugene's father.

Unhappily, Eugene's mood does not improve. After only three days he tells his parents that he is leaving again. When he and Arcady drive off in the tarantass, the old father is grief-stricken. But his mother, surprisingly and movingly, is able to comfort her husband. She tells him, 'A son is like a lopped off branch. As a falcon he comes and goes where he chooses; but you and I are like mushrooms growing in a hollow tree. Here we sit side by side without budging. But I shall stay with you forever and unalterably, just as you will stay with me.' Isn't that nice? She is not such a silly old creature after all. Turgenev is constantly surprising us by revealing new depths in his characters.

Back to Marino

So Bazarov and Arcady return to Marino, where Nicholas is still struggling to manage his estate and Paul is urging him to keep calm. But Arcady is still thinking about Nicolskoye and the two sisters. On a pretext of showing some old letters to Anna he gallops off there on his own and is very cordially received by both young ladies. This has the effect of getting him out of the way (and allowing his love life to develop) while matters between Eugene and Uncle Paul suppurate and come to a head. It all starts with Fenichka, for whom they are both harbouring amorous feelings. In one of their little chats together, Eugene invites Fenichka to smell some flowers and then surprises her with a kiss. She manages to push him off and reproaches him, but the scene has been observed by Uncle Paul, who feels that he must defend his brother's honour. He challenges Bazarov to a duel, which the young man thinks is absurd, but he coolly agrees to go through with it.

Pistols at dawn

The duel is atmospherically described and we really feel as if we, too, are in the field by the copse on that fresh, dewy morning, as the two adversaries grasp their pistols and pace out the distance. Bazarov still thinks the whole thing is absurd but he can't help wondering if he is going to die. Despite being a nihilist and a rude, insensitive one to boot, our Eugene conducts himself admirably. He is brave and unflinching as he sees Paul aiming at his nose and hears the sound of the shot. Then, without even aiming, he fires his own weapon and wounds Paul in the leg. The older man wants to exchange another shot, but Eugene won't have any more nonsense. In his role as doctor he takes control of the situation, bandages up his opponent's leg and makes sure that he gets back safely to the house. Fortunately the wound is not serious, and as soon as the patient is well again, Bazarov decides that, once again, it's time to move on. Uncle Paul has a new respect for him and wants to shake hands before he goes but, true to form, Eugene fails to show any warmth. After his departure, Paul seeks out Fenichka and establishes that she is truly and deeply in love with his brother Nicholas. He then urges his brother to marry her as soon as possible. So in a strange way, Bazarov's behaviour has enabled this to happen.

Love birds at Nicolskoye and other feathered friends

Meanwhile, over at Nicolskoye, Arcady is beginning to realise that it is Katya, Anna's unassuming but friendly little sister, whom he really loves. They have a number of tender scenes together. Finally, he starts working up to an awkward proposal of marriage 'while a chaffinch, perched in the foliage over his head, poured out its enraptured song'. Of course Katya accepts him, and I feel sure that two such nice and considerate young people will be very happy. With regard to that chaffinch, I must now tell you that this story is cooing and twittering with birds of every kind. Turgenev is clearly a bird fancier and he pops one in to act as a metaphor whenever he can. We have already seen Eugene compared to a falcon by his mother. When you read the book you will also discover a plump chicken (Nicholas?), a pigeon, a hawk (Bazarov again?), a greenfinch in a cage (Fenichka), a cock and a partridge, and probably others that I have missed. When Bazarov turns up and hears Arcady's good news, he points out a pair of jackdaws sitting side by side on the stable roof and says, 'There's a fine example for you! Take it to heart!' I didn't know this either, but apparently jackdaws are well known for their marital fidelity and belief in family values.

Bazarov goes home

So Arcady has chosen marriage and domesticity rather than the life of the rebel outsider. What will Bazarov do now? Anna invites him to stay longer, hinting that she might get over her fear of him. But Bazarov is not even tempted. Instead, he returns to his parents, who are naturally overjoyed to see him again. At first, he seems depressed and mopes about disconsolately. His mother tries her best to feed him and both parents fret about not being able to help, the way you do when a son or daughter is troubled and won't share it. Eventually, he cheers up and starts to help his father to provide medical services to the estate workers. The old man is really thrilled to have Eugene as his assistant; now his patients have access to all the latest scientific methods of treatment. But sadly, this is only a brief interlude. Tragedy is about to strike. Eugene performs an autopsy on a peasant who has died of typhus – and cuts his finger. Soon he becomes unwell, develops a high fever and has to take to his bed. Typically, he has no illusions about the prognosis. 'I'm in a bad way, old chap,' he tells his father. 'I've caught the infection. In a few days you will have to bury me.' The town doctor is sent for and various treatments are tried, without success. He asks them to send for Anna and she makes a dramatic appearance at his bedside, bringing yet another useless doctor. Anna and Bazarov have quite a touching final scene together. In his dying hours he reflects on his life and his imminent death. He sinks into a coma and a priest performs the last rites. And then the end comes. Although Bazarov has so often been rude, ungracious and annoying, I can't help feeling moved by the courage and honesty with which he faces his death. It's so sad that he is going to die before he has had a chance to sort himself out and use his gifts properly.

The epilogue

Instead of closing the book abruptly at this point, Turgenev allows his gaze to linger, so that we can see how his surviving characters will make out. First there is a double wedding: Nicholas and

Fenichka and Arcady and Katya are happily united. 'To Bazarov's memory,' whispers Katya to her husband as they clink glasses – and he gives her hand a squeeze. Anna eventually marries a lawyer (like Anna Karenina), 'a man still young and generous but also cold as ice. They live together in greatest harmony and may one day achieve happiness or even love.' And what about Uncle Paul? He has taken himself off to Dresden, where he may still be seen, cutting a distinguished figure on the terrace and in the salon. Finally, Turgenev's camera swoops down on a small, rather neglected village graveyard in a remote part of Russia. It is overgrown by weeds and the tombstones are all askew. 'Sheep wander at will over the graves. ... But in their midst stands a grave untouched by any human being, untrampled by any animal: only the birds at dawn perch and sing on it.' Ah, those birds again. I shall leave you to read this final paragraph for yourselves and, as you pay your last respects to the young nihilist, I shall not be surprised to see you brushing away a tear.

The text

Fathers and Sons by Ivan Turgenev was first published in 1862. I used an English translation by George Reavey, published by Hamish Hamilton in 1950 and purchased from the second-hand bookstalls outside the National Film Theatre in London. The translation by Rosemary Edmonds is available from Penguin books, and a more recent version, by Richard Freeborn, can be found in the Oxford World Classics series.

8

Strange Case of Dr Jekyll and Mr Hyde

by Robert Louis Stevenson (1886)
or
Dr Jekyll and Mr Hyde go to the movies

Brian Glasser

If everyone already knows a story, why tell it again? That may sound like a rhetorical question, but it does have at least two possible answers: one is that life's eternal truths need reiterating; another is that if you tell a story differently, it's not the same story anyway. With appropriate duality, both apply to the tale of Dr Jekyll and Mr Hyde.

The medium is the message

Let's address the second answer first: the simplest way to recycle a plot is to move it to a different medium. Artists do this all the time, lifting stories from the Bible for paintings, or from the theatre for operas, or from Greek mythology for poems. The land of literature is always being visited by movie-makers, usually using the bestseller list as their map – after all, half the advance publicity has already been done for these works. So it is hardly surprising that Robert Louis Stevenson's *Strange Case of Dr Jekyll and Mr Hyde* was turned into a film pretty soon after technology allowed, having been an immediate literary success when it was published in 1886. The success had, of course, been due to its startling subject matter, but also to its outstanding literary merits. For Stevenson was a deep-thinking writer who took pains over his craft – as a youth, in his own words, 'I was always busy to my own private end, which was to learn to write. I kept always two books in my pocket, one to read, one to write in'.[1] He brought his considerable skill as well as intellect to bear on the tale, which was therefore far more than a murder mystery or a Gothic pot-boiler – it was a brilliant rendering, in wonderfully measured prose, of the author's struggle with Calvinist conformism, the narrative permeated by silences, gloom and defeatism.

The first screen version appeared as early as 1908 and there have been many since – from the risible (*Abbott and Costello Meet Dr Jekyll and Mr Hyde* (1953), *Dr Jekyll and Sister Hyde* (1971)) to the respectable (Stephen Frears' and Christopher Hampton's *Mary Reilly* (1996)) – with an average of more than one every five years. Currently there is talk of a David Mamet-written and directed version to be called 'Diary of A Young Physician'. But whether high or low of brow, they are *all* grist to the myth-making mill.

By something approaching consensus, the best cinematic adaptation so far was made in the early days of the talkies, back in 1931. It could be referred to as the Rouben Mamoulian version, or the Fredric March version, or the Karl Struss version, or the Hoffenstein/Heath version, depending on one's particular interest – books (usually) have one author, but films are always the product of the efforts of many people. All the above were nominated for Oscars for their work on the film (except Mamoulian, who won a prize for it at the Venice Film Festival of 1932); and all were masters of their respective crafts, widely known in their time and still much admired by film aficionados.

Adaptation

To Samuel Hoffenstein and Percy Heath, the screenplay writers, fell the task of adapting the story in such a way that it would supersede previous versions. In the original, Stevenson had gradually heightened suspense by keeping the revelation that Jekyll and Hyde were one – if not one and the same – until the ninth and penultimate chapter, throwing in red herrings to keep readers' suspicions at bay. This was the climax of the book; and the explanation of the deeply disturbing phenomenon comprised the final-chapter coda – an exposition from beyond the grave by Jekyll himself, whose thoughts were at last revealed thanks to a letter he had left by way of posthumous apologia. The first eight chapters had been seen through the eyes of a curiously pallid bystander (a lawyer called Utterson).

In consequence, retaining the shape of the plot of the novella was not feasible – a whodunnit in which the murderer's identity is known in advance is a contradiction in terms, and a dull one at that. (Indeed, as a result of this, the book makes for a slightly curious read nowadays, its other qualities notwithstanding.) Furthermore, because knowledge of Jekyll's alias was withheld until the dénouement, causal analysis of his behaviour had been precluded until then too. So, paradoxically, while Hoffenstein and Heath were denied use of the original's trump card, a rich seam of creative opportunity was opened up to them – which they embraced with relish. Get rid of Utterson; get rid of the mists of mystery; and put Jekyll out in front from the off. He is the centre of attention from the first to the last scene of the film, and his character and attitudes are the basis for the whole of it.

Jekyll is shown in the first reel as a brilliant and charismatic doctor-cum-scientist who bridles at the limitations of the late-Victorian age. He gives a lecture at the academy, whose members are either appalled or patronisingly amused at his proposition that Man 'is not truly one, but two ... host to a good and a bad self'. A subsequent jousting match with his friend, the irretriev-ably staid Dr Lanyon, fills out this portrayal:

> *Jekyll: You have no interest in science at all. No dreams, no curiosity.*
> *Lanyon: There are bounds beyond which one should not go.*
> *Jekyll: Yes, it isn't done I suppose. I tell you there are no bounds, Lanyon. Look at that gas lamp. But for some man's curiosity we should not have it. And London would still be lighted by lamp boys. One day London will glow with incandescence. It will be so beautiful that even you will be moved by it.*
> *Lanyon: I find London quite satisfactory as it is. And I'm not interested in your short cuts and your byways.*
> *Jekyll: But it's in the byways that the secrets and wonders lie in science and in life.*

Smartly, Hoffenstein and Heath turn a problem – the audience's familiarity with the story – into an asset: they establish Jekyll's credibility at the lecture by actively using our prior knowledge (he *will* be Hyde, his bad self). They then reinforce this with a more objective, entirely unfictitious historical yardstick (electricity *will* be invented). Shortly afterwards, they enlist our sympathies as well, by showing him at work in hospital, where he tends to a needy charity patient in preference to going on a house-call to a hypochondriacal duchess. We are no doubt encouraged to side with Jekyll so that we feel his eventual fall the more keenly.

Enter the opposite sex. It might seem surprising now, in the early twenty-first century, but the novella included only the briefest reference to Jekyll's sex life (although sexual repression lurks behind the text's surface like a shadow) – it implied that he some-times visited prostitutes, as was not unusual for Victorian gentlemen. The 1931 movie was not the first adaptation to introduce the crowd-pleasing element of female pulchritude, but Hoffenstein and Heath judge their depictions of womanhood to a rare nicety. Jekyll's fiancée is the warm and attractive Muriel Carew. An early scene shows the pair sharing an easy-going rapport, as they slip out of a formal ball to share romantic badinage and a passionate embrace in the garden.

There's not much wrong with Muriel, but the same can't be said for her domineering father, a retired military man of the old school. There is more than a hint of male rivalry as the General repeatedly throws cold water over Jekyll's ardour; but his daughter avoids conflict in the steadfast belief that things will be all right in due course, a little patience being all that's required. This sanguine approach is more difficult for a man of Jekyll's temperament to adopt, and events proceed to make life harder rather than easier for him. While walking home with Lanyon from the Carews', he rushes to the rescue of a woman in the poor district who is being beaten up by a ruffian. It is a characteristic act, reflecting his spontaneity, his desire to right wrongs and his sense of duty as a doctor.

The victim's name is Ivy Pierson, and she turns out to be very attractive, although in a style somewhat different from Muriel's. Ivy is more sexually forward, and tries to seduce Jekyll in her room when she realises that he is handsome and well-to-do, and that his potential as a benefactor extends beyond the immediate circumstances. He draws the line at a kiss, which he laughingly says he will accept instead of a fee, but her overt sexuality has made an impression on him. As he walks away from the building with the disapproving Lanyon, Jekyll clashes with him about so-called respectable mores: he decries them as dishonest because they deny natural sexual instincts.

So the scene is set for the entry of Mr Hyde. Jekyll throws himself into his experiments instead of his love life, and finally arrives at a concoction which he believes will enable him to separate his good and bad selves. He drinks it in the interests of science – he writes a note to that effect in case he dies in the process – in what will prove to be his last heroic act. As he changes into Hyde, he scoffs at his doubters: 'Mad, eh Lanyon? If you could see me now ...'.

His butler disturbs him and he quickly drinks the antidote to turn back into Jekyll. Aware of the potential of what he has liberated, he renews his efforts to bring forward the date of his marriage to Muriel, but again the General rebuffs him. Muriel and her father soon depart for a spell in the country; and a few weeks later Jekyll receives a note informing him that her stay will be extended. His patience snaps, and he decides once again to assume the identity of Hyde – this time for a longer period, and this time with clear aims in mind. He visits the music hall that Ivy frequents, terrorises all and sundry (including Ivy), and soon has her set up as his kept woman at a flat in Soho.

Thus Hoffenstein and Heath make Jekyll's decision to drink the potion an understandable culmination of internal pressures in the face of an intransigent outside world – indeed it is a means of resolving some of these pressures. The first time he turns into Mr Hyde it is for science; the second is for sex, violence and unfettered self-expression. The frame of reference becomes firmly Freudian – 'Dr Jekyll and Mr Id' perhaps? – but that does not necessarily conflict with anything that Stevenson wrote (notwithstanding the fact that the book pre-dated the first publication of Freud's theories by ten years or so).

I am a Camera

Cinema was for many years looked upon by American intellectuals as infra dig, despite (or because of) the fact that it was flourishing as mass entertainment. It took the Europeans to call film 'the seventh art'. As such, its defining feature was the camera. Having given a little consideration to the work of the screenwriters, let us now look at the contribution of Karl Struss, the cameraman.

After a brief title sequence, the film opens as it means to continue – with arresting visual originality. The screen is filled with the forearms, hands and shadow of a man playing the organ – as seen from the position of the man's head. A voice is heard, and the camera tilts up and pans round to show a butler looking directly at, and speaking directly to, the camera. The organist (whom the butler has addressed as Dr Jekyll) is heard to reply, and then rises and walks through his opulent sitting room to the hall, where he is passed his hat and cape. We see all of this 'through the eyes' of Jekyll, in an extended use of subjective (or first-person) camera. There's a moment of cinematographic tension as Jekyll approaches a mirror in the hall to check his appearance – surely we'll simply see a reflection of the camera, surely this will

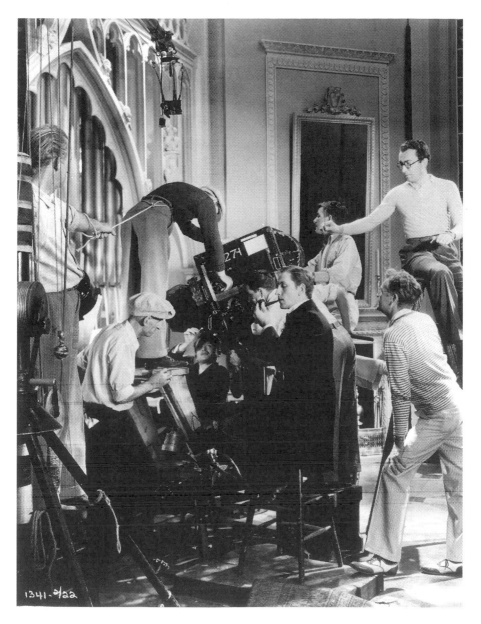

Film still 1
Director Rouben Mamoulian (far right, on ladder) lines up the opening shot of the film. Fredric March (Jekyll/Hyde) smokes his pipe while his musical stand-in plays the organ – note the latter's black jacket and formal cuffs. Karl Struss, the director of photography (in hooped sweater, beneath Mamoulian) supervises, while the focus-puller is held somewhat precariously by a rope.

signal the end of the uninterrupted Jekyll's-eye view we've had? Yet the expected cut never comes, and the camera continues to move until it is directly in front of the mirror – in which, somehow, we see the reflected figure of Jekyll! It's an exciting, purely cinematic moment, as well as being the perfect introductory view of a protagonist whose double-image is the subject of the film.

First-person camera was used in Hollywood before and after *Dr Jekyll and Mr Hyde* – think of the times you've seen an actor look out of the frame at something, followed by a shot of what he's looking at seen from his vantage point – but rarely in such a virtuosic manner. Struss was an American who had worked in 1927 with the great German director FW Murnau when the latter was in the US making a film called *Sunrise*. Murnau had presided over what remains one of the most celebrated subjective camera shots in cinema history (in *Der Letzte Mann/The Last Laugh* (1924)); and Struss has testified to the director's predilection for the non-stationary camera.[2] In the light of the opening sequence in *Dr Jekyll and Mr Hyde*, is it fanciful to suppose that such stylish practice was passed on from Germany to America like a baton in a relay race?

Dr Jekyll and Mr Hyde is packed with fabulous shots, and Struss clearly worked very closely with the set designer Hans Dreier to create a night-time London of half-lit alleyways and wholly felt unease. But his most famous contribution to the movie was in the scene where Jekyll turns into Hyde. In the reshaped plot, the transformation scene became a centrepiece of the film – and logically so, given its visual possibilities. Jekyll again stands in front of a mirror – this time in his laboratory – the better to observe the changes he will undergo. The subjective camera is also used again, and we see a beaker being tilted towards the lens as if to be drunk from, before the focus-puller adjusts what we can see to the previously blurred image in the mirror. A clever enough start, putting the audience right in the middle of the experience – but the best is yet to come. Without cuts or dissolves, we then watch Jekyll's face change over 20 seconds into the very different-looking Hyde's. In these days of computer-generated special effects, that would be unremarkable – but in 1931, it seemed miraculous. Its place in film mythology was ensured when absolutely no one would divulge how the feat of legerdemain had been accomplished – indeed it remained a secret for another 40 years! (Struss eventually explained that they had used coloured make-up on Jekyll and slowly removed like-coloured filters from the camera lens, a trick he'd tried out on an earlier movie which showed the healing of lepers! Full marks to actor Fredric March for his facial contortions too, which help make him unrecognisable as Hyde.) The camera then proceeds to whirl around, with various hallucinatory images coming in and out of focus, before we again see Hyde, who, with a couple of discreet cuts, attains his full appearance, sporting long hair and a false set of protruding teeth. Struss himself didn't like this vision of Hyde – 'They made him look like a monkey'[2] – and it is indeed an image that threatens contemporary viewers' suspension of disbelief. In fact, it was suggested more than once in the novella; and March pulls off a brilliant physical performance as Hyde; and there are several moments when Hyde's simian prowess is integral to the action.

Directions

Rouben Mamoulian is not among the best-known Hollywood directors. This is probably because he spent much of his time away from film-making, in the theatre – he was in charge of the first, ground-breaking stage production of *Porgy & Bess* – and because he was apparently unadept at the in-fighting required to prosper in Tinseltown. It is typical that one of his biggest hits – the very movie we are talking about – disappeared from circulation for almost 30 years less than ten years after it was made. Warner Brothers were making a new version starring Spencer Tracy and wanted to clear the field of competition. So – in what might be described as an act of Stalinist capitalism – they simply bought the distribution rights of the 1931 version from Paramount, put the film in a cupboard and threw away the key, thus effectively rewriting history (at least for a while). This was a testament to Mamoulian's achievement of course, and certainly the standard of much of his output is the equal of anything in the American cinema: *Love Me Tonight* (1932) is one of the most urbane musicals

ever made, and *The Mark of Zorro* (1940) is one of the most satisfying swashbucklers. The variety of genres he tackled may also
have militated against popular recognition, but there is a unity to
his oeuvre that is not apparent if you only look at storylines.

One writer has observed that 'One is ... tempted to say that
every Mamoulian film is a musical. It isn't true of course, but with
every action and every line of dialogue conceived in terms of
stylised rhythm – *choreographed* rather than directed – it feels as
though it were'.[3] This visceral effect of Mamoulian's movies is
part of his stamp, and so is his fearless attitude to film-making:
do everything the way it *needs* to be done, rather than how it's
been done by others. His boundless cinematic flair brings vitality
to every corner of *Dr Jekyll and Mr Hyde*, and when allied to the
intellectual sophistication that all his choices express, it explains
why an old and slightly crackly talkie remains so affecting. A
simple example is the first time that Jekyll presses for accelerated
access to Muriel's hand: the camera pans between two two-person
shots, one showing Jekyll and Carew, the other showing Carew
and his daughter. Only when Carew strides off unrepentantly
does Jekyll step into the space the General has vacated and bid
Muriel a fond, if desperately frustrated, good night. The visual
message, though understated, is clear – three into two won't go.
And this episode sets up the extraordinary one which follows shortly
after, where Jekyll rescues Ivy from her beating and helps her into
bed to recover. It is a scene of amazingly explicit sexiness which
would have been unfilmable a couple of years later when the
notorious Hays Production Code clamped down and took the
'sin' out of cinema in America. (In fact, several feet of film which
show (even more of) Ivy disrobing are still absent from the
version of the movie currently in circulation.)

Having accustomed the audience to the subjective camera in
the first scene, using it to get us to identify with Jekyll, Mamoulian
now deploys it to convey narrative material too: Ivy tells Jekyll to
look away so that she can undress for bed, and we see him turn
away (in a conventional third-person shot). But in the next shot
she takes off her stockings while smiling directly at the camera.
Because of the visual precedent, we read this as Jekyll having
turned back to look. This is confirmed when she throws her

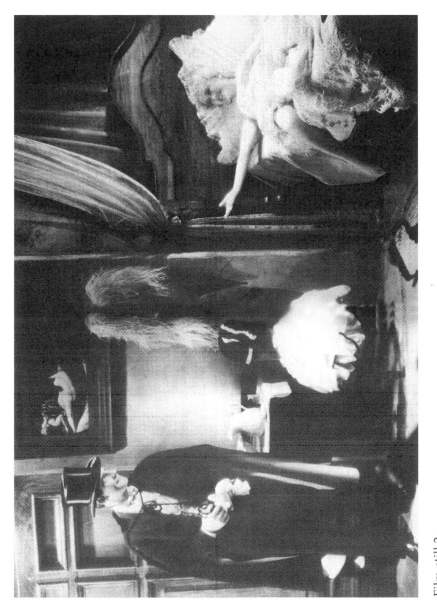

Film still 2
Ivy (Miriam Hopkins) invites Jekyll to come hither.

garters at the camera – Jekyll is heard to laugh and there is a cut to a shot of his shoes pointing in the direction of Ivy. In an unambiguous gesture, he places the tip of his cane in the middle of the circle of the garter. Later, as Jekyll walks home, thoughts of Ivy preoccupy him – there is an exceptionally long dissolve which keeps the fetching image of her naked leg swinging at the side of the bed on screen at the same time as we see and hear Jekyll conversing with Lanyon about sexual impulses and conventional morality (as described earlier).

This pair of Jekyll's encounters with women are thus presented very differently in an object lesson by Mamoulian in how to speak a fully integrated language of film, a language unlike anything that can be achieved in books or on the stage – we could also be noting in these scenes his sure handling of the acting perform-ances, the use (or relative absence) of dialogue, the careful choice of costume, and so on.

At a thematic level Mamoulian's sophistication is evident too – his entwinement of Hyde's sexuality with violence is eminently modern, as is Ivy's moth-to-a-flame masochism; and he discreetly nudges the study of Man's duality towards a contrast between nature and civilisation, instead of the more simplistic good and evil.

Fade out

Like most films, *Dr Jekyll and Mr Hyde* has imperfections that detract from its pleasures. But I shall let them pass like unhailed taxis; and allow readers to arrive at their own judgements when they see the movie. Best of all, catch it at a repertory cinema, where its visual delights can be fully appreciated. But in the meantime look out for its occasional screenings on television, or get hold of a VHS copy – it's available from America.

The Jekyll and Hyde myth is sometimes lazily conflated with that of Jack the Ripper, perhaps for reasons of temporal proximity. But while this is a false trail in its specifics – Hyde is not a pre-meditating serial killer, for instance – the recent evidence suggest-ing that the Ripper may have been the painter Walter Sickert does point to a fundamental similarity: that even the most outwardly accomplished and civilised of humans have rottenness inside them. This is the difference between *Dr Jekyll and Mr Hyde* – which was no doubt made at least in part to capitalise on the nascent horror-movie vogue – and the film of *Frankenstein* (released earlier in 1931), where the monster is an external creation of Man. The idea that we all have good and bad in us – or at the very least, civilised and brutish aspects – may nowadays be an accepted wisdom, not to say a banal observation; but that doesn't stop us experiencing feelings of remorse and disappointment when our behaviour errs on the uncivilised side. And here we find ourselves back at our starting point: eternal truths.

The distance between eternal truth and cliché is often small, and to be measured in how a story is told rather than what it is about. This 70-year-old treatment of *Dr Jekyll and Mr Hyde* is an utterly absorbing hour and a half of cinema, an enduring and endearing work of art.

The text

Stevenson RL (1886) *Strange Case of Dr Jekyll and Mr Hyde*. Longmans, Green, London.

References

1   Stevenson RL (1887) *Memories & Portraits: IV – A College Magazine*. Chatto & Windus, London.

2   Higham C (1970) *Hollywood Cameramen*. Thames & Hudson, London.

3   Milne T (1969) *Mamoulian*. Thames & Hudson, London.

Further reading

•   Anobile RJ (ed.) (1975) *Film Classics Library: Dr Jekyll & Mr Hyde*. Avon Books, New York.

On-screen credits: *Dr Jekyll And Mr Hyde* (Paramount, 1931)

Directed by Rouben Mamoulian
Screenplay by Samuel Hoffenstein and Percy Heath
Photographed by Karl Struss
Cast

Fredric March	Dr Henry Jekyll / Mr Hyde
Miriam Hopkins	Ivy Pierson
Rose Hobart	Muriel Carew
Holmes Herbert	Dr Lanyon
Halliwell Hobbes	Brigadier-General Carew
Edgar Norton	Poole, Jekyll's butler
Tempe Piggott	Mrs Hawkins, Hyde's landlady

Thanks are due to Warner Brothers for their permission to use the film stills in this chapter.

9

The Death of Ivan Ilyich

by Leo Tolstoy (1886)

Now I would like to tell you about one of Tolstoy's most celebrated short stories. In *The Death of Ivan Ilyich*, he describes how a prosperous and self-satisfied lawyer develops a nagging pain, which remorselessly progresses to become a terminal illness. Just before he dies he reflects on the emptiness of his life and undergoes a profound spiritual change. Because of its theme and Tolstoy's brilliant portrayal of the sick man, the story is often used in medical humanities courses for doctors and medical students in the hope that it will help them to learn something about the feelings of dying patients and the effect of terminal illness on the rest of the family.

In the first volume of *Medicine and Literature* we discussed the wonderful *Anna Karenina*, which Tolstoy finished in 1876. Now you might expect *Ivan Ilyich*, written ten years later, to have similar qualities, and to some extent it does, especially as the great man's skills in bringing his characters to life (and, in this case, to death) were undiminished. However, in those ten years Tolstoy had undergone a terrific emotional and spiritual upheaval; he had become disgusted by what he saw as a total lack of moral purpose in his own life.

He came to believe that he had lived only to satisfy his urges (mainly sexual) and to lead a rich, comfortable life on his country estate. Even his books served no purpose except to win him the admiration of other writers. He no longer believed in God and so his life seemed pointless. At first he wanted to commit suicide but he felt too scared. The crisis was resolved when he came to the conclusion that God did exist after all, and that what he needed was the simple unquestioning faith of the Russian peasant rather than the elaborate ritual and doctrines of the Orthodox Church. And so the great novelist became the founder of a religious movement which had followers all over the world. Basically, he believed that everyone ought to live a good life in accordance with the teaching of Jesus. For Tolstoy this meant no sex (or as little as possible, even in marriage), no violence, giving up one's possessions and living in poverty. He described the crisis and the changes in his inner life very powerfully in a short work called *A Confession* (1879). After that he tended to think that writing fiction was vain and sinful, and tried to give it up. But every so often the imaginative writer would escape from under the cloak of the prophet. When *The Death of Ivan Ilyich* appeared in 1886, his readers must have been delighted to have a new story from the pen of the old master. But how much has his 'conversion' affected the way he writes? Let us look at the story and see for ourselves.

The death is announced

As the story opens we find ourselves in the Law Courts of St Petersburg where a group of lawyers are discussing a case during a break in proceedings. One of them, a man called Piotr (Russian for Peter) Ivanovich, is idly looking through the *Gazette* when he is shocked to discover the announcement of the death of their colleague Ivan Ilyich Golovin. When he tells the others, they don't seem particularly bothered. They knew he had been ill but they hadn't realised it was serious. They will have to go and pay their respects to his widow, which is a bit of a bore. But Tolstoy also tells us that, privately, they are all speculating about how the vacancy left by Ivan's death will affect their own chances of promotion. The other emotion they all share is a complacent pleasure that: 'it is he who is dead, and not I'. Not a very nice bunch, are they? But Piotr Ivanovich has decided that he must go and see the widow that same evening, so perhaps he is a more decent fellow than the rest.

Piotr drives off to Ivan's house where people are gathering. He follows the others into the room where Ivan's body is lying in state, according to the Russian custom. He notices the servant, Gerasim, strewing something on the floor and he becomes 'instantly aware of a slight odour of decomposing body'. He gazes at his dead friend's face, which looks handsome and impressive but also reproachful. Outside in the hall he has a few words with his friend Schwartz, who makes it clear that their regular whist game will go on as usual that same evening, in spite of Ivan's no longer being available to take a hand. Tolstoy keeps letting us know that Ivan's friends will not allow his death to interrupt their normal pleasurable activities. Do we hear the heavy irony of Tolstoy the prophet? I think we do.

But Piotr is not going to be joining the card players just yet. The widow has taken him by the arm and is leading him off to the drawing room for a talk. She tells him about the last three days and nights of her husband's life in which he screamed for hours on end. The suffering of his old classmate fills Piotr with horror – after all this might happen to him too, without any warning. But again, he is consoled by the thought that it had happened to Ivan and not to him; and cheerful thoughts about life dispel fearful ones about death. The widow then gives him a long account of her own suffering (which he finds rather wearisome) and goes on to ask his advice about 'how she could obtain a grant of money from the government'. Piotr attends a brief service round the body of the dead man and observes Ivan's son, who looks just like his father. His eyes are red with weeping, although he has the look of 'nasty minded boys of thirteen and fourteen'. It's all very depressing and Piotr escapes with relief. He arrives at the card game just in time to join in the second rubber, and that is the last we see of him.

A brief survey of Ivan's life

'The story of Ivan Ilyich's life was of the simplest, most ordinary and therefore most terrible.' With this arresting sentence Tolstoy begins the second chapter. And so we survey this ordinary life and wonder what will make it so terrible. Ivan is the son of a government official and he grows up to be 'an intelligent, polished, lively and agreeable man'. As a law student he does some things which make him feel disgusted with himself (don't we all?), but when he finds that other people of good standing are doing them too, he stops bothering about it. He takes his degree and gets a good first job as a minor civil servant. He has a few affairs and a few drinking bouts and a few 'after-supper excursions to a certain outlying street', but again he is no different from his well-bred friends. He becomes an examining magistrate and enjoys the power that this position gives him over people's lives. He meets a suitable young woman, Praskovya Fiodorovna; she falls in love with him and he says to himself, 'After all why not marry?' Is he in love with her? Well, maybe a little, but mainly he marries her because it would be looked on as 'the correct thing'.

The couple's happiness is short-lived. Once she is pregnant, his wife becomes jealous and demanding, and starts to make 'disagreeable, ill-mannered scenes'. When their first child arrives, their relationship gets more distant. Ivan decides to insulate himself from his tedious domestic life by concentrating his mind on his work. From now on he will require from his married life only 'a wife to manage his house, meals and a bed'. He and Praskovya have more children (two of whom die) and the usual ups and downs of married life, but they continue to quarrel bitterly. There are only occasional 'rare periods of amorousness', which are like 'little islets at which they put in for a while, only to embark again on a sea of hostility'. Ivan spends less and less time with his family.

Eventually, with a little help from an influential friend, Ivan lands a prestigious post as a judge. Now he can move back to the centre of the fashionable world in St Petersburg and enjoy a salary of 5000 roubles a year. Even Praskovya is pleased at the news. Ivan goes off to the city by himself to find a set of suitably impressive apartments and to have them furnished in the lavish style that he can now afford. He rushes around buying furniture and choosing decorations. He even assists the workmen in hanging up curtains and has a minor fall off a stepladder in which he bruises his side. When all is ready, his wife, son and daughter join him in St Petersburg and his new life as an important person begins. He settles into a pleasurable office routine. Tolstoy makes a point of telling us that while his dealings with his clients and petitioners are always correct, he likes to keep the human side of these relationships to the absolute minimum. Ivan is really pleased with his professional success and he enjoys relaxing over a game of whist with his cronies. He and Praskovya move in the best circles and are well thought of in society: but they are not happy. They continue to quarrel violently.

What is Tolstoy up to?

Now I would like to pause and take a look at what Tolstoy, the master storyteller, has been doing to us in this account of Ivan's life. There are several things about it that disturb me. The first is that, unlike in *Anna Karenina* and *War and Peace*, he has given us a principal character who is really not at all sympathetic. Ivan is greedy, self-centred and mercenary; he hates his wife and cares nothing for his children. He seems to be without a single spark of human warmth and decency. And yet, Tolstoy has cunningly made us believe that we are under his skin, feeling everything with him. How did he make us empathise with someone so cold and unpleasant? And why did he choose such a person for a 'hero'? There is, it seems to me, a resemblance between Ivan and one person in *Anna Karenina*, and that is Anna's husband, Alexei Karenina. He is also a self-important official and a cold fish; but there are times when he has our sympathy and concern. The second thing I notice about Ivan's life is that his moral shortcomings are exactly the same as the ones for which Tolstoy chastised himself so severely in *A Confession*. And yet, for us, the most distressing aspect of Ivan's life is the way he ignores his wife and children. If we were to ask Tolstoy's own long-suffering wife, Sofya, she would tell us that, as a husband, he only became really insufferable and arrogant *after* his 'conversion'.

So the great man's view of himself is not very reliable.

Ivan starts to feel unwell

Now we must return to Ivan Ilyich, who is beginning to feel unwell. The illness begins with 'a queer taste in his mouth and a sort of uncomfortable feeling in the left side of the stomach', in much the same area that he injured in his fall from the stepladder. He becomes more irritable, domestic rows occur more frequently and Praskovya is heard to say that her husband has always had a dreadful temper 'and that it had needed all her good nature to put up with it for twenty years'. Again, Sofya Tolstoy would have said, 'exactly like my husband'. Eventually Ivan's wife realises that he is physically unwell and she persuades him to consult a celebrated doctor. I am sorry to say that the physician in question is not very patient-centred. In fact, his professional manner is rather like that of Ivan himself when dealing with a prisoner in the dock. He sets out the diagnostic possibilities and weighs up the evidence, but doesn't tell Ivan whether or not his illness is 'serious', which is the one thing he wants to know. He only tells him that his pain is probably due to appendicitis – although it could be due to a 'floating kidney'. Let us not bother too much about these two outmoded diagnoses: no doubt, with the onward march of evidence-based medicine many of our own favourites will be out of fashion in another 100 years.

Looking for a cure

On the way home, Ivan keeps going over the doctor's words in his mind, the way patients do. When he gets home he tries to tell his wife and daughter about it, but they are much too preoccupied with planning their own lives. Ivan tries to take his medicine regularly and follow the doctor's advice. He becomes gloomily interested in other people's accounts of their illnesses and compares them with his own. When he has an upset at work, or even at cards, the pain gets more intense. He blames his bad luck, or even the people who have angered him, for making his condition worse. He reads medical books and consults other doctors. He finds himself almost believing a story about a miracle cure involving an icon. And all the time he is feeling worse and worse. The pain in his side nags away, his appetite is poor, his breath seems to smell bad. Poor old Ivan, I feel really sad for him now. He is so lonely and terrified. Meanwhile, Praskovya takes the view that it is all his own fault. She tells her friends that he simply won't follow the doctor's advice: he forgets his medicine, eats the wrong food, won't rest and so on. He continues to go to the courts and to play cards with his friends, but it is becoming an increasing strain. Why, he wonders, is everyone one else so well and cheerful?

The truth begins to dawn

One day, his brother-in-law comes to visit. When he sees the deterioration in Ivan's appearance he is visibly shocked. And so are we, because this is the first time we have been told that he looks emaciated. Ivan overhears him talking to Praskovya in the next room. She thinks he is exaggerating but he says: 'Why, surely you can see for yourself – he's a dead man! Look at his eyes – there's no light in them. But what is it that is wrong with him?' Praskovya replies that nobody knows. Even the doctors disagree.

Ivan walks away and thinks about the floating kidney. In his mind, he tries to catch it and make it firm. He goes to see yet another doctor who tells him it's his appendix; but with the right treatment, its functioning can be regulated and restored to normal. 'Secretion and evacuation' need to be re-established. Is it all just due to constipation? In bed that night (he sleeps alone in a separate room now) he feels that the appendix is improving already. Then the horrid pain returns. Suddenly he realises that it's not just a question of appendix or kidney. He really is dying. I guess he must have an abdominal cancer, maybe of the stomach or colon. He is so lonely and frightened as he lies there, I feel a tremendous compassion for him, even though he is such an obnoxious chap and I would never choose him for a friend. He is terrified both of dying and of being dead. He rages against all the healthy people who are 'making merry'. Death will come to them soon as well. In his agitation he starts to panic and get breathless. He knocks over the bedside table and his wife hurries in. She asks what is the matter, and calls him 'Jean', a pet name, which she doesn't often use. She suggests getting a specialist to do a home visit. Ivan refuses and she kisses his forehead. Tolstoy records that 'He hated her from the bottom of his soul while she was kissing him.' Oh, God, this really is 'terrible'. Where is the palliative care team? Where the marital therapist and where the friendly, understand-ing family doctor?

Ivan is alone with his thoughts, as he has been for so long. He thinks about his happy childhood. He was always such a special little person. Surely he wasn't meant to die, just because it's well known that everyone has to die. He goes into a phase of denial and tries to carry on at work, ignoring the pain. But even as he presides in court, the pain won't let him alone. It seems to stand before him and look at him. At home he tries to distract himself by tidying up his beautiful sitting room. He tries to put up a mental screen to keep out the pain, but *it* keeps peeping through. Is this how it really feels to know that you have a fatal illness? Is this how our tiresomely obsessive hypochondriacal patients feel? Will we too share Ivan's experience one day, if we don't avoid it by stepping under a bus?

The patient takes to his bed

We are now in the third month of Ivan's illness. He now seems to be too weak to leave his room. He is having opium by mouth and morphine injections, and although the pain is less intense he feels drowsy and uncomfortable. The only person he can tolerate is his servant Gerasim, a cheerful, straightforward young peasant lad. Gerasim helps him to go to the toilet and cleans him up without making him feel embarrassed at being so helpless. Ivan likes to rest his legs on Gerasim's shoulders and talk with him. Now the family and the doctors are treating him as an invalid, but they all keep up the pretence that he is going to get better. We doctors have all seen this and perhaps felt we had to share in the deception for fear of upsetting everyone (including of course ourselves). But Gerasim is more open and honest. When Ivan tells him he can go to bed and rest himself, Gerasim says it's no trouble to stay and look after his master: 'We shall all of us die, so what's a little trouble?' For Gerasim, death is not a forbidden subject. The other thing that upsets Ivan is that there is nobody to pity him. He would like to cry on someone's shoulder and be comforted like a child. But his stern attitude to his family and friends makes this impossible. In this respect he is not like the average dying patient, who can at least accept the love and care of those close to him. But he is a bit like a stubborn old novelist/prophet called Leo Tolstoy.

And so Ivan waits for death in constant anguish. He makes the occasional effort to take control. He has a wash and brushes his hair. Then he catches sight of his face in a mirror and 'his heart went cold at what he saw, especially at the limp way in which his hair clung to his pallid forehead'. A cup of tea makes him feel better for a while – but soon the pain and the bad taste return. The doctor comes to call. He is a hearty, cheerful fellow who rattles on about the weather. When Ivan tries to tell him about the pain, he hardly seems to listen. After the examination, Praskovya joins them and complains to the doctor about her husband's non-compliance with the treatment regimen. Later on (at Praskovya's behest) a specialist arrives and examines Ivan again. He and the GP have an earnest discussion about whether the kidney or the appendix is at fault. When Ivan looks up at him timidly and asks if there is any chance of recovery, the great specialist answers that 'he could not vouch for it but there was a possibility'. This is the point where we physicians are supposed to encourage the dying patient to express his deepest fears, and if he is ready to hear it, to tell him the truth. But this is not going to happen. The doctor departs and after another injection, Ivan falls asleep. He awakes to find his wife all dressed up to go out to the theatre. His daughter Lisa and her young man are going with her and they too come into the sickroom. Lisa seems to her father to be wonderfully strong and healthy and in love – but also 'impatient with illness, suffering and death because they interfered with her happiness'.

His son, little Ivan, the schoolboy we noticed at the funeral, also appears. He is the only one who shows signs of distress at his father's condition: but they do not exchange any words and there is no physical contact. The theatregoers leave, not wanting to be late, and Ivan is once again left alone with his pain and his anguished thoughts.

Ivan reviews his life

I say he is alone, but we readers share everything with him: the tedium, the sweating fear, the anger and the misery. I can even feel the pain and taste the taste. Tolstoy may have become a terrible, bigoted moralist but, when the wish to write a story returns to him, as occasionally it still does, he has lost none of his ability to make his readers feel they are actually living in the world he has created.

Now, on his deathbed, Ivan starts to weep and to rail against God, at His cruelty, at His absence. I think we have all been there once or twice. Then he hears a voice within him, perhaps the voice of his soul, asking 'What is it you want?' He replies that he wants not to suffer, but to live 'pleasantly' as he used to do. And then he starts to review his life from the beginning (much as Tolstoy had done in *A Confession* a few years earlier). His recollections of his childhood are pleasing; but the further he gets from childhood the less good he is able to find in his life: his marriage, his career, 'that deadly official life and the preoccupation with money' all seem to have been worthless and senseless. And now he has to die. He becomes more and more agitated. Could it possibly be that he has not lived as he should have done? But no, he has always done his duty, so that is impossible. He is not yet ready to accept the awful truth.

More weeks pass. Ivan lies on his sofa, in his bleak, lonely state. Now he feels that he is falling into a black abyss; the only bright spot is his childhood far behind him. Ahead, as he falls like a stone, with increasing velocity, there is only increasing pain and misery culminating in death. Another fortnight passes. His daughter Lisa has got engaged to her boyfriend and Praskovya would like to tell Ivan the good news; but his condition has taken a turn for the worse. When his wife and daughter come in and ask how he is, his only response is to say, coldly, that 'he would very soon relieve them all of his presence'. The doctor says that his sufferings must be truly terrible, but Tolstoy tells us that his mental torments are now far worse than the physical pain. Last night he looked at Gerasim's good-natured peasant's face and realised with a shock that his life has indeed been wrong all along. He has conformed to the way of life prescribed by the highly placed people he admired and suppressed all those 'scarcely noticeable impulses' to fight against it. All his adult life, domestic, professional and social, has been 'a monstrous lie'; his position is totally indefensible and it's too late to do anything about it.

Ivan's life: 'most ordinary and therefore most terrible'?

Before we get totally carried away by Ivan's sickening realisation, we might make our own assessment of his life. Has it really been so bad that he deserves to make himself suffer like this? As lawyers go, he is surely no worse than thousands of others. And if he had only been a little more considerate of his wife's feelings and allowed his own humanity to breathe more freely, he and his family would have been much happier. OK, he hasn't been a saint, but he is not a criminal either. The trouble is that for Tolstoy, reviewing his own life, if you weren't a saint (and a severe, intolerant, cantankerous saint) you were more or less a moral criminal. At least, that's how he felt about himself and so he inflicted the same stark alternatives on Ivan. It's also worth remembering that Tolstoy concluded in *A Confession* that the only person who really knew the right way to live was the Russian peasant, with his supposed simple, sturdy faith. Hence the presence of Gerasim as both an ideal comforter and a demonstration of all that Ivan has failed to be in his own life.

The end is near

Whatever we think of Ivan's self-appraisal, the last chapter has an awesome and uplifting power. It is quite short because Ivan has not much time left. He has dismissed everybody except Gerasim from the sickroom and now he starts to scream in agony for three days and nights. He feels as though he is being forced, struggling, into a black sack, by an unseen, invincible power, perhaps an executioner. He can't get out, but neither can he get completely into the black hole. 'What hindered him from getting in to it was his claim that his life had been good.' Suddenly a blow in the chest forces him through: 'he sank through the hole and there at the bottom was a light'. It's like being reborn. Suddenly he is more peaceful: ' "No it was all wrong," he said to himself, "but no matter." He could, he could do the right thing. "But what was the right thing?" he asked himself, and abruptly grew quiet.' A moment before, his little son had come in and seen his father's distress. He puts his hand on the boy's head. The boy kisses his father's hand and bursts into tears. Somehow poor Ivan finds little Ivan the easiest person in the family to respond to, perhaps because he reminds him of his own child self. His wife comes in too, with tears on her face, and he feels sorry for both of them. He tries to ask for forgiveness but the word comes out as 'forego'. 'Everything oppressive' now seems to be falling away from him; the fear of death has completely gone and has been replaced by light. Ivan is at last at peace. It takes another two hours for his heart to stop but the spiritual agony is over. To the considerable relief of the reader, who has been suffocating in the black hole along with him.

Remembering Ivan

I feel tremendously moved by Ivan's death but I have lots of questions and I expect you will have too. Is that what death will really be like? Is it true that you can't die until you have accepted that your life was all wrong? And if so, is a terminal glimpse of the right way to live enough to provide redemption? And what sort of redemption? Is Tolstoy telling us that Ivan has now gone to Heaven? Personally I can't accept that line of thought. But it makes me wonder what dying patients are thinking about as they lie there, veiled by morphine. Can good palliative care protect a dying patient from all the agonies that Ivan has to suffer before he gives in? We can relieve physical pain, in most cases, but what about the spiritual pain? Perhaps people need help to see that their lives have not been so bad after all. I don't think many people get the opportunity to review their lives with a friend or a doctor or a minister before the end. On the few occasions when I have been able to do this with a patient, it has always felt right.

I think we should definitely keep reading *The Death of Ivan Ilyich*, painful though it is. Having immersed myself in it for a week, I am sure I shall remember it every time I enter the bedroom of a dying patient. It may even help me to have the courage to say: 'Now that it's nearly over, what sort of a life do you think you have had?'

The text

The Death of Ivan Ilyich by Leo Tolstoy, first published in 1886. An English translation by Rosemary Edmonds is published by Penguin. Extracts reproduced by permission of Penguin Books Ltd.

Further reading

A Confession by Leo Tolstoy was first published in 1879.

There is a good modern biography, *Tolstoy* by AN Wilson, published in 1988 and now available in a Penguin Classic Biography edition.

Postscript: What's so terrible?
Tolstoy's art of dying by Alistair Stead

The contemporary American novelist Stanley Elkin has proposed that two elements go into the making of fiction: the learned and the inspired. About inspiration in the case of Tolstoy's novella, I shall have a word or two to say shortly. But it is the learned aspect which seems at first to be most apposite in the context of *Medicine and Literature*; for prominent in Elkin's list of those tried and true traumas for the generation of narrative interest which most writers of fiction may inherit and learn from literary tradition is 'bad news from the doctor'. This virtually archetypal situation of the modern era may go some way to justifying the narrator's claim that the story of Ivan's life (and death) is 'most simple and ordinary'. I shall return to this not-so-simple issue after I have addressed another.

You will notice that I have chosen to call *The Death of Ivan Ilyich* a novella rather than a short story, as John has called it. If I followed John's preference I would myself have written 'long short story' in any case, as a modest warning to readers. My immediate and favourite access to an English translation of this great work is, as it happens, a superb anthology of six Russian short novels selected by Randall Jarrell, an American poet and critic with an unerring instinct for spotting (literary) winners. I don't want to make too much fuss about defining with a show of pseudo-scientific precision the genre or literary kind to which this story belongs. To condense a cautionary saying of the French poet Valéry, you don't get drunk on wine labels. Nevertheless, my strategy would be to use the term novella (or short novel) to evoke the original meaning of both terms, since they derive from the Italian *novella* ('a tale, a piece of news'). Hence the rightness of reminding the reader that everything depends on introducing into the life of Ivan some new thing: 'bad news from the doctor'? No, *terrible* news. News about something that will enable us to recognise how Ivan's life has been 'most terrible'. (And it is terrible news for doctors, too, with its savage caricature of the medical profession!)

Curiously enough, my own experience of reading outstanding novellas tempts me to generalise rashly and state that, for no immediately obvious reason, they have, in a variety of ways, been great vehicles for terror, terrifying fables. Humour me a moment while I reel off a few instances: Heinrich Kleist's *Michael Kohlhaus*, Henry James's *The Turn of the Screw*, Dostoevsky's *The Eternal Husband*, Thomas Mann's *Death in Venice*, Ivan Bunin's *The Gentleman from San Francisco*. Even the gentle Chekhov, often seen as the antithesis to Tolstoy, was capable of nightmare visions ('But perhaps the universe is suspended on the tooth of some monster') and produced his appalling *Ward 6* – definitely a candidate for Dr Salinsky's special treatment. These are in addition to the examples of the novella which John has been introducing to you in this volume: Conrad's *Heart of Darkness* and Kafka's *The Metamorphosis*.

And it is not just male-authored texts engaging subtly with the exotic materials of the historical, the Gothic or the decadent kind that bring you naught for your comfort. I can recommend a whole line of novellas by women, especially by American women writers, which in spite of, or maybe on account of, their often conventionally domestic settings, can terrify just as much: try Edith Wharton's *Ethan Frome*, or Willa Cather's *My Mortal Enemy*, or Katharine Anne Porter's *Noon Wine*, or Tillie Olsen's *Tell Me a Riddle*, or Joyce Carol Oates's *Black Water*. Still seeking to justify my hunch about the novella, I might point to the sacrifice in them of extensiveness to intensity of effect, and there are, in a phrase George Steiner has used to characterise Tolstoy's achievement in *Ivan Ilyich*, 'the violent energies of compression'.

So, in considering the art with which Tolstoy handles the process of dying, and the time-honoured sensation, *Timor mortis conturbat me* (Latin for 'Fear of death throws me into confusion'), I should like to risk a little rather technical study of what Randall Jarrell has called 'one of the most frightening sentences in literature', the challenging sentence which opens the second section of the story and to which I have already alluded: 'The story of Ivan Ilyich's life was of the simplest, most ordinary and therefore most terrible.' This is Rosemary Edmonds's translation of the Russian: '*Proshedshaia istoria zhizni Ivana Ilyicha byla samaia prostaia i obyknovenia i samaia uzhasnaia.*' Hers is in at least one respect superior to the pioneering and still widely available Aylmer Maude version which begins with 'Ivan Ilych's life was ...', because it stresses, as the initial phrase of the Russian does (literally, 'the past history'), that the life is something being told in a certain way, presented to us as a story, which happens to be 'most simple'.

But I prefer, as you see, Maude's 'most simple' as more direct, closer to the literal translation of the original, to Edmonds's rather quaint 'of the simplest', which introduces a variation where the text prepares for the hammer blow repetition of 'most' in 'most terrible'. 'Most simple' can be understood as indicative both of the commonplaceness of the events that make up Ivan's life and of the form or style of its narration. This appears to accord with Tolstoy's later articulation of his artistic credo: 'The business of art consists precisely in this, to make intelligible and accessible to all what might be unintelligible and inaccessible in an intellectual form.' Yet the story transcends this somewhat simplistic aesthetic doctrine, since, although the story comes across impressively at one level as a satirical fable, a relentless exposure of the society of which Ivan is a typical product, the technique is always more sophisticated than at first appears. For instance, notice how this conjoined 'simple' (as accusation of unthinking mediocrity) is picked up near the end of his life by Ivan and charged with positive value as he approaches enlightenment, at last showing some concern for others: 'How good and how simple!' (The sound of the root syllable of the Russian for 'simple', 'prost', also seems to be echoed with ironic force when a humbled Ivan tries to utter 'forgive [me]', 'prostitye', but produces only 'forego', 'propusti', for he/everyone must relinquish this life, particularly the life lived badly, before forgiveness, which crucially includes self-forgiveness, is possible.) There may also be a suggestion of how a certain *simplification* in Ivan's story occurs because he has deliberately shrunk the scope of his own actions, chosen to live, from an ethical point of view, reductively, in following the constricting logic of his worldly pleasure-seeking milieu.

Here it is perhaps useful to look both backwards and forwards in Tolstoy's canon, comparing his fictional treatment of the dying. If we look back to *War and Peace* (1869), we find that the last days of the wounded soldier Prince Andrey, who has reconciled himself to inevitable death, passed 'in an ordinary and simple way', that is, as they should. He makes a good death, surrounded by family, having received the last rites and duly blessed his son. In the famous sentence in *Ivan* the intensifier 'most' (in Russian, *samaia)* yokes together 'simple and ordinary' as if to propose how close, virtually identical, they are in meaning and so sets them off that much more startlingly against 'most terrible'. (The Bernard Guilbert Guerney translation which Vladimir Nabokov approves, melodramatises this by introducing 'and therefore most terrible' with a dash.) This insinuation of the paradoxical nature of the hero and his fate recalls the opening of Kleist's marvellous early nineteenth-century *Novelle, Michael Kohlhaus*, where Kohlhaus is slightly more obviously set up as a conundrum for our contemplation: 'one of the most upright and *at the same time* [*zugleich*] one of the most terrible men of his day' (my emphasis).

Although Ivan has an epiphany at the close, dropping self-pity, recognising the virtue of the devoted service and clear-eyed compassion of the young peasant Gerasim, and acknowledging the suffering and needs of others (his wife and son), so that his own pain and fear of death are suddenly abolished, his death falls short of the self-sacrificial death in a later novella of Tolstoy's, the still impressive *Master and Man* (1895), where what is a psychological turning point for Ivan, the merest *impulsion* to do 'the right thing', to lose his shallow self-centredness, is, in accord with that late turn towards didactic art, converted now into an exemplary *action.*

Reversing in a brilliantly realised crisis the conventional roles of master and servant, Tolstoy makes the death of the former in a tremendous snowstorm enable the survival of the latter. The dying merchant loses all terror in the joy of his effort to save his hard-drinking labourer from freezing to death and is given knowledge thereby of 'the real thing'. All three accounts of dying men appear to be inspired by the writer's own experiences. He had a never-to-be assuaged anxiety about death, what it might usher in or open onto. (Since he was plainly a brave soldier and an intrepid hunter, it was not a matter of the terror inspired simply by the prospect of physical pain and dissolution.) But he also had enjoyed a near-death experience, which gave him authentic insights to enable the superb rendering of Prince Andrey's narrow escape from annihilation in the Battle of Austerlitz and the servant Nikita's awakening from the deepest chill. What Tolstoy had not experienced of course was death itself, and his observational powers and compelling imagination do wonders with the plausible presentation of dying moments. His skilful deployment of a virtual stream of conscious technique in all three instances suspends disbelief, both by its attention to minute particulars in the circumambient world of the dying and by the stark, hallucinatory imagery which haunts the expiring man (the black sack or hole, the sound of a voice calling one's name).

Remarkable as is Tolstoy's power to evoke our final moment, he stops at the threshold of any revelation of an afterlife. Christian though he is and possessed of missionary zeal, he tends to withhold pious reassurances. After Prince Andrey dies, his sister asks in vain, 'Where has he gone? Where is he now ...?' Ivan has his vision of light displacing the blackness of death, but no more than that, and we have already witnessed the tawdry aftermath of his death in the devastating overture to the story, full of incomprehension, hypocrisy and self-deception on the part of the survivors on whom his death appears to have had no moral impact. Even in the more orthodoxly oriented *Master and Man*, with the master's dying cry of 'I'm coming' and the peasant's prayer to God before his seemingly imminent death, we are immersed in a very down-to-earth rendering of sensation and scene, and the story ends with only a shadowy notion of that 'other life' beyond the servant's actual, very ordinary demise. For, as has been noticed before, the title of Ivan's story is a misnomer (or at least incomplete): it is in essence, as the terrible sentence says, about the life, not the death, of a man. Tolstoy's religious vision of how his character approaches the end of his life combines both the old attention to the *moment* of dying (is it a good death?) and the new tradition of seeing the end as a final judgement on a *whole life*.

Here one might take note of the inspiration. We may trace, as John has done very reasonably, the seeds of the novella back to the morbid self-analysis in *A Confession*. But something came from further outside himself, helping him, I would contend, to escape idiosyncrasy. In 1881 he had read about the death of a public prosecutor with a very similar name to the one in the story: Ivan Ilyich Mechnikov. The change of surname to Golovin would suggest that Ivan acts too calculatingly (*golova* means head); he lacks heart (sincerity, passion, compassion). This is, then, as he names the topic for his projected tale, essentially about 'the death of a judge', one whose important occupation becomes the passing of sentences and one on whom a more terrible sentence has been passed.

At first, Tolstoy had Ivan tell his own story in a diary passed on to us by a colleague, so the parallel with *A Confession* would have been closer, but the shift to the third person establishes a judicial distance from the subject, allowing for a broader indictment of the society in which the shallowness of the judge has flourished: hence the part played by Piotr, that Ivan-to-be. Something of the original design remains in the artful organisation of the published tale: there is the tripartite structure of the posthumous action, handled dramatically by scenes; then the first part of the flashback devoted to reporting Ivan's career often in summary fashion; then, the application once more of the intensely dramatic method to scenes of Ivan's drawn-out agonies, but coloured by his tortured vision. Where we have more of the narrator's external view, in the first and second parts, we can see without Ivan's complacent blinkers how bleak is his habitat. Yet the third part allows us to see that it is not all terrible. He dies in bed at home. We can see Gerasim, even if he is idealised, bringing selfless comfort. We can see, at last, the credible weeping of the son and wife. Contrast the lonelier end of an updated, socially reduced Ivan, an overreaching and dissolute Hollywood talent agent, dying without friends or family, with only an anonymous nurse in attendance in the characterless ward of a Los Angeles hospital, as pictured in Bernard Rose's 2002 movie *Ivansxtc*. Furthermore, what surpasses cinema's external view is the increasing intimacy in print of an imaginative penetration into the dying Ivan's perspective which can bounce us into belief in the fact and force of the instant of death itself, and more: we can overhear, perhaps longingly, surely compassionately, that silent voicing of Ivan's triumphant self-consolation ('"Death is finished," he said to himself. "It is no more."'), an illusion perhaps, but one which the great illusionist's art may have made us momentarily at home in. For fear of worse?

Further reading

Stanley Elkin's distinction between the learned and the inspired appears in the Preface to his anthology of *Stories from the Sixties* (Anchor Books, 1971), which includes *Tell Me a Riddle*. *Master and Man* (translated by Nathan Haskell Dole) appears together with *The Death of Ivan Ilyich* (translated by Aylmer Maude) in *Six*

Russian Short Novels selected with an Introduction by Randall Jarrell (Anchor Books, 1963), which also includes *Ward 6*. For details of the genesis of Tolstoy's great novella, a convenient summary appears in David Magarshack's Afterword to the Signet Classic edition of *The Death of Ivan Ilyich and Other Stories* (The New American Library, 1960).

10

Heart of Darkness

by Joseph Conrad (1902)

When I first tried to read Conrad I found him very difficult and had to give him up. I knew that he was a highly respected author of sea stories and I was attracted to the title *Lord Jim*. I think maybe the name 'Jim' reminded me of Jim Hawkins of *Treasure Island* and I was expecting a rollicking tale of a boy hero's adventures with rascally pirates. But Conrad's way with words is very different from Stevenson's: I got all tangled up in the rather convoluted narrative and had to abandon ship. I did read *Lord Jim* many years later when I had more patience, and found it very enjoyable. But before that I discovered *Heart of Darkness* in a different way. I went to see the Francis Ford Coppola film *Apocalypse Now*, which was based on the Conrad story. If you have seen it you will remember that it is set in the Vietnam war and that Marlon Brando gives a blood-curdling performance as an army officer who has been left in charge of an isolated outpost a long way up river and has gone crazy. When the rescue party reaches him they discover that he is being treated by the locals as a kind of god-king, loved and feared and executing anyone who displeases him. The chaos of the Vietnam war clearly has a lot to do with his moral breakdown, but we are also led to believe that he has had some piercing insights into his own soul and the human capacity for evil.

Impressed by the film, and always interested in literary sources, I tracked down the book (which, thankfully, did not have Marlon Brando on the cover). It was surprisingly small, only 111 pages, and I didn't think it would occupy me for long. In this I was mistaken for several reasons. First of all, as with my first attempt on *Lord Jim*, the writing slowed me down. I had to keeping pausing because the images were so vivid, and because some of the phrases kept echoing in my mind and giving off different meanings. Then I frequently found myself uncertain about what had actually happened in the story: Conrad's narrative texture is not transparent – the story is about an expedition into the jungle and the words seem like rich thick vegetation which you have to examine carefully as you thread your way along. So I read it quite slowly, going back over the bits that puzzled me. Then I read it again. By the time I had read it the third time I was beginning to get the hang of it and was really enjoying myself, savouring the words, the sounds and the smells. I do hope this is not putting you off: I will try to act as your guide through the jungle – but we are not going to use a machete because the jungle is too mysterious and beautiful to destroy. The whole book is almost a poem.

Who was Joseph Conrad?

Let's begin with a few words about the author. The two things you may remember about him from school are that he was Polish and that he was a merchant navy officer before he became a writer. His name was originally Józéf Teodor Konrad Korzeniowski, and he was born in 1857 in a part of the Ukraine which was then culturally Polish but ruled by Russia. His parents both died when he was a young boy, and his guardian was his maternal uncle. Young Konrad loved reading sea stories and was determined to go to sea himself. He persuaded his uncle to let him go and stay with some relatives in Marseilles, who were in the shipping business. Soon he was learning to be a sailor, first as an ordinary seaman (a very tough life) and later, after studying and passing his exams, as a ship's officer. He liked English ships best, and rapidly learned to speak the language. In 1890, Conrad accepted an assignment to take a small steamer up the Congo to supply a remote trading post. This experience was later used as the basis for *Heart of Darkness*. He suffered badly with malaria and dysentery in Africa and that was more or less the end of his sea-going career. He had already published his first novel (*Almayer's Folly*) and he decided to hang up his sea boots and become a captain of English prose. Everyone marvelled (and we still do) that a man with such a thick Polish accent could write such wonderful English. He married an Englishwoman called Jessie George and they had two children, but there is not much about love and sex in his books. He was quite a private man and we don't know very much about his inner life – only what he tells us indirectly in his novels.

Heart of Darkness

So now I think we are ready to start on our journey up the Congo with Joseph Conrad. The story begins on the Thames estuary, somewhere near Gravesend. The sun is just beginning to set, and a little group of friends are sitting on the deck of a boat (a cruising yawl for those of you who know one kind of ship from another) called the *Nellie*. The company consists of the author himself, the director of companies, the lawyer, the accountant and a seasoned sailor called Charlie Marlow. Marlow is the only one who still 'followed the sea', and while they are waiting for the ebb tide to float them off on their cruise, he entertains them with a story (which in fact takes up the rest of the book, once it gets going). Conrad uses this Marlow character as his narrator in several other books, including *Lord Jim*. He seems to be a sort of alter ego who allows Conrad to talk about his own memories and emotions at one remove and at a safe distance. In this book Conrad describes Marlow as having 'sunken cheeks and a yellow complexion' – probably how he looked when he himself returned from the Congo, ravaged by malaria 12 years earlier.

Before handing over his narrative to Marlow, Conrad gives us a magical description of sunset over the wide, placid waters of the Thames estuary. He imagines the historical English seafaring heroes, such as Francis Drake, setting off for fame and fortune on the same tide. What wonderful inspiring fellows he seems to say; how proud we are of them. But when we read the book a second time we wonder if he is being ironic: weren't they really just self-serving, murderous pirates? Dusk falls, and we watch the lights on the river. Then Marlow with one of his arresting utterances suddenly says: 'And this also ... has been one of the dark places of the earth.' Everyone listens and hangs on his words. He goes on to sketch a picture of the Romans arriving in Britain 1900 years earlier. For these 'civilised' men, used to a comfortable life in Rome, Britain must have seemed like a wilderness: cold, foggy, disease-ridden and dangerous. Those nice young Romans in their togas, he says, must have shivered with fright as they looked at the ancient British 'jungle' surrounding them.

> Land in a swamp, march through the woods and, in some inland post, feel the savagery, the utter savagery, had closed round him, – all that mysterious life of the wilderness that stirs in the forest, in the jungles, in the hearts of wild men ... And it has a fascination too that goes to work on him. The fascination of the abomination – you know, imagine the growing regrets, the longing to escape, the powerless disgust, the surrender, the hate.

When I read this passage the third time, I realised that it was a kind of overture to the whole work: a summing up of what happens when a group of people try to take over a country that doesn't belong to them. But even on a first reading of *Heart of Darkness* you quickly realise what Conrad feels about imperialism:

> The conquest of the earth, which mostly means the taking it away from those who have a different complexion or flatter noses than ourselves, is not a pretty thing when you look into it too much. What redeems it is the idea only.

So what is the 'idea'? Marlow seems to be making a concession towards the beliefs of his listeners that the creation of a colonial Empire was a noble enterprise bringing civilisation, law and order, education, Christianity and trade to the poor ignorant natives. But his story rapidly undermines the credibility of that version as we shall see.

Marlow reminds his friends that he once 'did a turn as a fresh water sailor for a bit' – and they know that they are in for one of his long and 'inconclusive' stories. He begins by telling them of his boyhood desire to explore the blank spaces on the map of the world. Most of them had since been coloured in, but the centre of Africa still fascinated him. No longer 'a white patch', it was now 'a place of darkness' with 'a mighty river that resembled an immense snake uncoiled, with its head in the sea, its body at rest curving afar over a vast country and its tail lost in the depths of the land'. The prospect is alluring and also threatening; but there is no stopping Marlow now. We are in for a trip up the snaking river into the heart of darkness.

The preparations

In the next few pages, Charlie Marlow relates how, with the help of an influential old aunt, he found himself a job with a continental company which trades on the river. Since the river was the Congo the company must have been Belgian. His assignment is to take command of a river steamboat whose previous captain has been killed 'in a scuffle' with a native chief over a couple of hens. There is a chilling little account of this incident, which is a warning of things to come. At the time, however, Marlow is not put off – he is only too pleased to have the opportunity of taking over the command of the steamer. There are some tedious formalities to go through in the company's offices, including a medical examination. As usual, when a doctor appears on the scene, we must pause and see what he has to say. This doctor is an elderly man whose research interest (or perhaps it's just a hobby) is to measure the cranium of those going out to Africa. He never sees them when they come back so he is not able to repeat the measurement but in any case 'the changes take place inside, you know'. He advises Marlow at all costs to stay calm when in the Tropics; irritation, he says, is even more dangerous than exposure to the sun. More warnings, but our hero is not deterred. He goes to say goodbye to his aunt, who gives him the last cup of tea he is to enjoy for many months and cheers him on his way with a few imperialist sentiments: 'She talked about "weaning those ignorant millions from their horrid ways", till, upon my word she made me feel quite uncomfortable. I ventured to hint that the company was run for profit.'

The journey begins

At last we are off! Isn't this exciting? After all those frustrating delays and tiresome debates about morality, the boys' adventure story is at last beginning. Marlow sets off for Africa in a French steamer which calls at various ports round the continent. As the African coast slips by, he is intrigued by the sights of the jungle and by the thought of the mysteries lying inland. 'Come and find out', the coast seems to be saying. At one point they come across a French warship which is anchored off the coast and firing shells into the bush in an apparently blind manner. 'In the empty immensity of earth, sky and water, there she was, incomprehensible, firing into a continent .... There was a touch of insanity in the proceeding.' The explanation is that 'the French have one of their wars going on'; but the image of the gunboat blindly shooting up Africa stays in your mind as a symbol of imperialist insanity.

Thirty days later, Marlow reaches the mouth of the river and changes to another steamer, which will take him upstream. After 30 miles, they reach the first of the company's trading stations. What are they trading? We don't know yet, but the vibrations are not good, are they? Marlow's first impression, as he steps ashore, is of decay and dilapidation. The first thing he sees is a boiler 'wallowing in the grass', suggesting that steamships don't do well here. He also observes a railway truck lying on its back and some other pieces of discarded machinery. Then 'a slight clinking made me turn my head'. It is the sound of iron chains and collars around the necks of prisoners. In another example of his brilliantly effective command of English, Conrad/Marlow shows us a pathetic group of Africans, chained together and slowly climbing a hill under the supervision of an armed white guard. The prisoners are thin and out of breath. The guard grins at Marlow and seems to regard him as a confederate. 'After all,' Marlow tells his listeners with heavy irony, 'I also was a part of the great cause of these high and just proceedings.' But actually he is horrified. He has seen all sorts of devils in men: the devils of violence, greed and hot desire: but this imperial devil seems to be something worse – 'a flabby, pretending, weak-eyed devil of a rapacious and pitiless folly'.

Even worse sights will soon appear to sicken him (and us). He comes across a group of emaciated Africans who are clearly dying 'as in some picture of a massacre or pestilence'. We are not clear what has happened to them and one can't help being reminded of pictures of Africans dying of famine or AIDS. We watch as one of the dying men crawls painfully towards the river to drink. Suddenly a white man appears in a high starch collar, white cuffs, natty jacket and white trousers, and varnished boots. He is carrying a green parasol. This is the company's chief accountant, coming out of his office to get 'a breath of fresh air'. Marlow has to wait at the station for ten days with only the accountant to talk to – but from him he hears for the first time about a man called Mr Kurtz. If you have seen *Apocalypse Now* you will remember that Colonel Kurtz is the Marlon Brando character who becomes seriously disturbed in the Vietnamese jungle. All we learn about the original Mr Kurtz at this stage is that 'he is a very remarkable person'. He is in charge of the furthermost trading station up river and he sends in as much ivory as all the others put together. *Ivory*! So that's what this trade is all about! One of those over-valued commodities like gold and diamonds, which notoriously inspire greed, theft and violence. 'Mr Kurtz will go far, very far,' says the accountant importantly. We may suspect that Mr Kurtz may have already gone much too far, but that discovery remains in the future.

To the Central Station

The next stage in Marlow's journey into the darkness (and towards Kurtz) is a 200-mile hike across country to the 'Central Station', where he will reach the river again and take command of his steamer. He has one European companion and 60 African bearers, who, I suspect, have to carry the white men in litters as well as all the luggage on their backs. (Conrad has a distressing tendency to refer to Africans as 'niggers' but, given his general lack of racism, I think that he was following the usage of his time and not meaning to be offensive.) The Central Station is on a backwater surrounded by scrub and forest. Marlow is dismayed to learn that his precious steamer is lying at the bottom of the river as a result of an ill-managed attempt to take her upstream two days earlier. The next few months are occupied with fishing the wrecked boat out of the river and attempting to repair her with the inadequate means available. Marlow gets down to it quite happily – he is always in a better mood when he has work to do and can get his mind off the monstrous crimes his fellow Europeans are committing in Africa in the name of progress. He also learns more about Mr Kurtz from the manager of the station. There have been rumours that Mr Kurtz is very ill; that his whole station is in jeopardy. The manager is 'very, very uneasy'. He is anxious for Marlow to get the steamer afloat and get down to Kurtz as fast as he can in time to avert some sort of catastrophe. Other white men who are hanging around at the Central Station also contribute to Marlow's gradually accumulating stock of information about Kurtz. One impresses on Marlow that Mr Kurtz is an important and enlightened man who will soon be promoted to an important administrative post in the company.

Also waiting for the boat to be repaired is a group of newcomers, Europeans, who are keen to get into the interior where they can get involved in the ivory trade. They talk about it constantly: 'The word "ivory" rang in the air, was whispered, was sighed. You would think they were praying to it. A taint of imbecile rapacity blew through it all like a whiff from some corpse.' Marlow refers to these chaps contemptuously as 'the pilgrims'.

The rumble in the jungle

Eventually the repairs are finished and the ship's ancient boiler gets up steam. We are on our way again, up the river to find out the truth about Kurtz. If you want to picture the boat, it is a paddle-steamer, with a single large wheel at the stern. The boiler is at the front and behind that are two little wooden deck houses.

The whole thing is covered by a light roof on stanchions. The funnel sticks up through the roof and in front of it is a small cabin which acts as pilot house. Our crew consists of 20 Africans (whom Marlow describes rightly or wrongly as 'cannibals' or 'savages'). We are also carrying the pilgrims, the hopeful ivory traders, as passengers. There are memorable descriptions of the scenery: 'Going up that river was like travelling back to the earliest beginnings of the world, when vegetation rioted on the earth and the big trees were kings. On silvery sandbanks, hippos and alligators sunned themselves side by side.' Has Conrad's imagination run away with him a little there? And wouldn't they be crocodiles in Africa? No matter, we are spellbound and tense with anticipation. What will be waiting to greet us round the next bend? Occasionally there are glimpses of villages through the dense foliage. We hear yells and even glimpse the inhabitants: 'a whirl of black limbs, a mass of hands clapping, of feet stamping, of bodies swaying, of eyes rolling, under the droop of heavy and motionless foliage'. But mostly the 'tin pot steamer' just crawls slowly along – towards Kurtz.

Fifty miles from our destination, the Inner Station, there is a derelict hut of reeds where Marlow finds a tattered old manual of seamanship. Outside the hut is a pile of wood and a notice saying: 'Wood for you. Hurry up. Approach cautiously.' A couple of days later, as the sun rises, a dense white fog envelops the river. From out of the dense jungle, now quite close, comes 'a very loud cry of infinite desolation' followed by terrifying shrieks and screams which seem to come from all around. The hostility is palpable. 'Will they attack?' whispers somebody. The Europeans are all tense and frightened. The Africans seem to find it merely interesting. The headman offers to eat their opponents if Marlow can catch them. Marlow observes that they have brought with them only a lot of disgusting decayed hippo meat and they must be very hungry. He wonders why they don't simply kill and eat the five white men.

There is no time to think about that any more because the boat has now entered a narrow channel, not very deep and too close to the bank. A shower of little sticks whizzes from the shore, falling on the boat. Then, a few lines later, we realise that they are arrows! This is one of Conrad's specialities: a slight delay before the full shock-horror is revealed. The 'pilgrims' start shooting wildly into the trees. The African steersman, in a panic, opens the shutter of the pilot house in order to fire a big rifle – a fatal mistake, as he gets a spear through his chest. His death is vividly described in Conrad's best boys' adventure story style. In the end the natives are scared off by a trick of Marlow's, which I am reluctant to reveal (all right, he uses the steam whistle). Then he tears off his shoes (which have filled up with the dead man's blood as it flowed over the deck) and flings them overboard with disgust. He feels despair at the thought that Kurtz is probably dead too and he will never get to talk to him. At the memory of this, Marlow breaks off his narrative, and demands some more tobacco for his pipe; we suddenly remember that we are not in Africa but in England, on the entirely peaceful deck of another little ship anchored in the Thames.

A meditation on Kurtz

The excitement of the attack on the steamer is over; we have reached page 68 (just over halfway) and you will, by now, have some idea of how such a small book can provide such a long and satisfying read. Marlow now changes gear and shifts forward in time. He did get to meet Kurtz and he wants at this point to tell us about the man. This is a rather strange way of ordering his book and you might think it would make more sense to continue the story chronologically; after all, now the fight is over we are minutes away from stepping ashore at the Inner Station. But that is not Conrad's method. He wants to describe Kurtz before Marlow meets him. So Marlow begins to reminisce about Kurtz and we realise that he has been very impressed, and not altogether negatively. His appearance was impressive to begin with – his bald head was like a great ball of ivory. And Marlow seems to have spent a long time listening to Kurtz talking about himself and his ideas. Kurtz had written a 17-page report for the International Society for the Suppression of Savage Customs – but that was 'before his – let us say – nerves, went wrong, and caused him to preside at certain midnight dances ending with unspeakable rites'. The report is full of noble and benevolent ideas – although it does recommend that Europeans should take advantage of the fact that the Africans will tend to regard them as gods. Nevertheless, it is beautifully written and Marlow is moved by its eloquence. But he is dismayed to find that, at the foot of the last page and at a later date, the degenerating Kurtz has scrawled in an unsteady hand: 'Exterminate all the brutes!'

The last days of Mr Kurtz

After expressing his ambivalent feelings about Mr Kurtz (severe disapproval mixed with admiration and wonder), Marlow picks up his story at the point where he throws his shoes overboard. We have reached Kurtz's station at last. Through his binoculars, Captain Marlow can see a hill with a decaying building at the summit. Near the house are half a dozen slim posts 'their upper ends ornamented with round carved balls'. The remains of a fence? I don't think so. I want you to remember those posts because we shall get a closer view of them shortly. While the others go ashore and prepare to enter Kurtz's house, guns at the ready, Marlow stays on the boat and talks to a young Russian seaman who is Kurtz's admirer and, it seems, his last disciple. He tells Marlow about life with Kurtz and how the 'simple people' loved him and how he had great plans for them. But on the other hand: 'He could be very terrible. You can't judge Mr Kurtz as you would an ordinary man.' Looking again at the house through his glasses Marlow now has a closer view and sees that the 'round carved balls' on the posts are in fact *human heads*. Ugh! Although still under the spell of Kurtz's charisma, Marlow has to admit that Kurtz 'lacked restraint in the gratification of his various lusts'.

When they enter the house Kurtz proves to be very ill indeed. They carry him on a stretcher to the boat and put him to bed in the cabin. Shortly after he is installed 'dark human shapes' emerge from the forest. Two warriors in fantastic headdresses take up a stand by the river. Then 'a wild and gorgeous apparition of a woman' begins to move towards the boat as if coming to reclaim

Mr Kurtz. Fortunately, she turns aside at the last minute and disappears into the bushes. From his couch in the cabin of the steamer, Mr Kurtz continues to protest that they are stealing his ivory (large quantities of which have been discovered and piled on board). He insists that he will return and 'carry my ideas out yet'. One can't help agreeing with the manager who tells Marlow that 'his method is unsound'.

During the night Kurtz summons his strength for a desperate escape bid and crawls off the boat in an attempt to rejoin his ghastly followers. But Marlow courageously goes after him and drags him back on to the boat, still arguing. Back in captivity Kurtz continues discoursing in his eloquent voice. He talks about his 'Intended' (his fiancée back home), his station, his career, his ideas, but also about the wealth and fame which he thinks are still waiting for him. Gradually, as the boat steams back downstream, Kurtz's strength fails. He clearly has malaria and possibly dysentery as well. Near the end 'a change came over his features I have never seen before'. Marlow wonders if he has reached a supreme moment of self-knowledge. And finally: 'he cried out twice, a cry that was no more than a breath – "The horror! The horror!" '

Those words echo in Marlow's mind – and in ours too. Back in England he has to go and see Kurtz's 'Intended' and break the news to her of his death. Conrad tended to regard women as rather sacred beings who lived in a special world of their own in which they must not be disturbed. When he meets Kurtz's fiancée, Marlow has a difficult time. She, of course, is expecting to hear only praise of her beloved. Marlow, surprisingly, says that he knew Mr Kurtz 'as well as it is possible for one man to know another'. He finds himself tacitly agreeing with her that Kurtz was his friend and that it was impossible, if you knew him, not to love him. He has a nasty moment when she asks what were Kurtz's last words. He can almost hear them being whispered aloud: 'The horror! The horror!' Then, in a moment of inspiration, he tells her a lie: 'The last word he pronounced was – your name.'

Trying to reach a diagnosis

What really happened to Mr Kurtz? Did he have a psychotic breakdown? He certainly has some features of a bipolar disorder. He has delusions of grandeur, he is obsessed by unrealistic projects, he is intolerant of any criticism. There are also hints of periods of profound depression. I can imagine myself going into that house with a social worker (trying not to look at the heads on the posts) and doing a mental health assessment. Should Kurtz have been 'sectioned'? There was certainly ample evidence that he was likely to do harm to others, so I think they were right to remove him with a view to compulsory observation and treatment. It's just unfortunate that his physical health was even worse than his mental health.

Alternatively, should we really think of him as evil? There were certainly some very nasty things going on in his mind resulting in some unspeakable acts against the people who trusted him. But Marlow/Conrad is also at pains to let us know that there was an inspirational side to his character as well; indeed, he has been described by a colleague as 'an emissary of pity and science and progress, and devil knows what else'. So what was it that drove him over the edge and made him give way to the dark side of his nature?

Was it prolonged exposure to the 'savage' ways of the tribal Africans? Contemporary readers might have thought so and Conrad himself talks of witch doctors and cannibals. But we who have seen the savagery that 'civilised' Europeans are capable of, are less likely to think that so-called primitive people are more prone to murder each other than we are.

Another possibility is that the whole colonial, imperial enterprise, with its thinly disguised greed and brutality, will tend to coarsen and brutalise anyone who gets involved in it, especially if he finds himself in a position of unlimited power. There is plenty of evidence that this happens and we can see from reading *Heart of Darkness* how strongly Conrad felt about it.

And finally, in addition, there is the inner psychological explanation which Marlow himself urges upon us. Here was a man who looked into the depths of his own soul and saw in his own 'heart of darkness' the evil of which man is capable. He struggles with it, but in the end the evil or the madness overcomes him. He loses control and at the very end of his life all he can see is 'The horror!'

In a stunning last paragraph, Conrad returns us to the listeners on the deck of the *Nellie*. The director observes that they have 'lost the first of the ebb' while they were absorbed in Marlow's story. And Conrad, in his own voice tells us that:

> The offing (the way to the sea) was barred by a black bank of clouds, and the tranquil waterway leading to the uttermost ends of the earth flowed sombre under an overcast sky – seemed to lead into the heart of an immense darkness.

Your turn

And now it's time for you to read *Heart of Darkness* for yourselves. It's a short book, as I keep saying. But it will stay with you for a long time.

The text

Heart of Darkness by Joseph Conrad was first published in serial form in a magazine in 1898–99. It appeared in book form in 1902, along with *Youth* and *The End of the Tether*. *Heart of Darkness* on its own is now available from Penguin Books.

11

The Metamorphosis, The Burrow and *Josephine the Singer*

Three animal stories by Franz Kafka (1915–24)

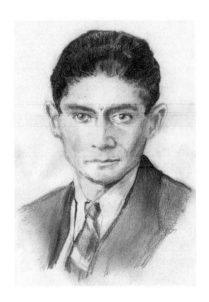

The first volume of *Medicine and Literature* opened with my enthusiastic report on Kafka's short story *A Country Doctor*. Now we are going back to Kafka to have a look at some more of his brilliant, enigmatic stories, in particular the ones featuring animals. Was Kafka an animal lover? I don't think he ever kept one as a pet, but in his stories he often seems to imagine himself as an animal with human feelings and aspirations. We are going to look at three of these stories, in which the featured creatures are respectively a beetle, a mole (or is it a badger?) and a singing mouse. We'll begin with the beetle.

The Metamorphosis (1915)

Part I

This is one of Kafka's best-known works and probably one of the best short stories ever written. This is how it begins:

> *As Gregor Samsa awoke one morning from uneasy dreams he found himself transformed in his bed into a gigantic insect. He was lying on his hard, as it were armour-plated, back and when he lifted his head a little he could see his dome like brown belly divided into stiff arched segments on top of which the bed quilt could hardly keep in position and was about to slide off completely. His numerous legs, which were pitifully thin compared to the rest of his bulk, waved helplessly before his eyes.*

At first, Gregor thinks it must be a horrible dream or at least some temporary state which will soon revert to normal. Well, you would, wouldn't you? But after a while he realises that his transformation is permanent. Is Kafka writing a totally bizarre horror story, which could never happen to any of us in real life? I don't think so. This must be what it feels like to wake up with some devastating illness like a stroke, and gradually to realise that you and your body will never be the same again. Gregor is a young man, I would guess in his late twenties, and he works hard as a salesman. Today he has overslept and his chief worry is about getting to work without catching a reprimand from the chief clerk. His mother and father and sister all call to him from adjoining rooms asking why he doesn't get up and whether he is unwell. Of course they can't see him yet and so he can persist in the unrealistic belief that his life can carry on as before. The world hasn't really changed, it's just a matter of getting the hang of how to work this cumbersome, unfamiliar, insect-type body. But it's not easy. Gregor has a terrible struggle getting himself out of bed and figuring out how to coordinate all his little legs. How many does he have? There should be six if he's an insect but we get the impression there could be a dozen pairs. In any case a beetle on his back has a major problem in getting his feet on the ground again. Again, I can see parallels with the plight of patients and remember being unable to get out of bed myself when I had a lumbar disc prolapse.

Unlocking the door

Eventually the chief clerk himself arrives to find out why Gregor has failed to turn up for work. (Even that is a pretty horrifying minor nightmare: imagine your boss turning up outside your bedroom door when you have slept through the alarm.) The door is locked, Gregor can't yet get to it and they all think he is refusing to open it. Trying to pacify them, he calls out: 'I'm just going to open the door this very minute. A slight illness, an attack of giddiness, has kept me from getting up.' If only it were true. If only the stroke or the disc or the cancer had never happened and the symptoms were genuinely trivial. But his attempts at reassurance only increase the agitation of those outside the door. For one thing they can hardly understand him, his voice no longer sounds human. I need hardly remind you that stroke patients may have similar problems with their speech. Eventually, with the aid of a chair Gregor manages to lever himself up on end and attack the door key with his mandibles, doing them some damage in the process (ouch). When he finally edges himself round the door the effect is, of course, devastating. The chief clerk backs away in horror, his mother collapses and his father knots his fists then 'covered his eyes with his hands and wept till his great chest heaved'. Gregor tries desperately to communicate with them, to explain and to reason with them. He gets his feet on the ground and discovers that he can walk really well on those little legs of his. His mother springs to her feet, backs into the table and knocks the coffee pot over. When poor Gregor smells the coffee he can't resist snapping his jaws together and that throws everyone into a complete panic. The chief clerk flees in terror down the staircase as Gregor's father picks up his stick and drives his insect son back into the bedroom. In his haste to comply Gregor gets stuck in the doorway and injures his side. The first part of the story ends with his father brutally shoving him back in and slamming the door shut.

Part II

The story is divided into three equal parts like a three-act play. In part II we see Gregor trying to come to terms with being a beetle and to renegotiate his relationships with his family. Through the closed door he listens to them discussing their problems at meal times. They are now hard up because, since the failure of his father's business a few years earlier, Gregor has been supporting the family with his salary. He had even been hoping to pay for his sister Grete (who plays the violin) to go to the Conservatory. At first Grete seems to be kind and helpful. She is not afraid to enter Gregor's room and she provides him with a choice of different foods to see what will appeal to him. Gregor discovers that old cheese, stale bread and rotting vegetables are what he likes best. Fresh food is a complete turn-off for a beetle. Then he discovers that it can be great fun to scamper up the walls and hang suspended from the ceiling where he can breathe more freely. Sometime he loses concentration and falls to the floor but is unharmed. Life as a beetle has a few compensations. To spare his sister's feelings he always hides under the sofa when she comes into the room with his food. After a while, his mother decides that she would like to visit her son also. When this has been achieved (with Gregor out of sight), Grete persuades her mother that it would be best to move out all the furniture to give him more space. When Gregor sees what is happening he is very upset. He is particularly anxious not to lose a picture of a lady dressed in furs, which hangs on one wall of his bedroom. So he protects it by clinging to the glass in the frame. When his mother catches sight of 'a huge brown mass on the flowered wall paper', she screams and collapses onto the sofa. Then everything accelerates towards the disaster.

Grete rushes out to get smelling salts, Gregor follows (trying to help), gets cut on a broken bottle and, in his agitation, starts crawling randomly to and fro over the furniture, walls and ceiling till he falls on to the table. Then his father returns and pelts him with apples, driving him once again back into his room. One of the apples sticks in his back causing a painful injury. The last thing he sees as the door closes on him again is his mother pleading with his father to spare their son's life.

Part III

This is the final act of the tragedy – or is it a bizarre comedy? Gregor is now a disabled beetle and a very sick one as a result of the rotting apple embedded in his flank. He is still spurned by the family but they open his door in the evenings to allow him to listen to their conversations. His father has taken a job as a bank messenger and wears his braided uniform all the time. Gregor lies thinking about his old life and dreams of once more taking charge of the family finances. His sister Grete has become fed up with taking care of him and scarcely bothers to clean his room any more. Gregor has lost his appetite and scarcely eats any more: he is clinically depressed as well as injured.

Meanwhile, to supplement their meagre income the family have taken in lodgers, three strange bearded men who share a room and like everything to be scrupulously tidy. One evening, Grete plays the violin to them all in the sitting room. Gregor listens and is entranced by the beauty of his sister's playing. 'Was he an animal,' asks Kafka, 'that music had such an effect on him?' This is very sad. He crawls forward hoping to pull at the skirt of Grete's dress and draw her into his room to play for him. The lodgers spot him, and once again there is a horrified reaction to Gregor's presence in the sitting room. He tries to return quickly but once he is back in his room with the door slammed, it is clear that it will soon be curtains for the unhappy beetle. The lodgers give in their notice. Grete, his dear sister, proposes that they get rid of Gregor at once. She now refers to her brother as 'it' and declares that 'it' can't really be Gregor. If he had had any human feelings he would have gone away of his own accord. Again, I think of a seriously ill patient, who perhaps has disgusting smells and distressing habits due to brain deterioration. His family are beginning to think he would be better off in a nursing home. For his own good, naturally.

But Gregor is already dying. And when he eventually slips away the family undergo a kind of regeneration and revival of their energy and zest for life. There is no mourning period whatsoever – they are shamelessly glad that their embarrassing, metamorphosed former son and brother has been tipped onto the rubbish heap by the helpful charlady. This is a little hard to take for us readers, who are genuinely fond of Gregor. Perhaps it reflects Kafka's morbid (and almost certainly inaccurate) feeling that his own family would be glad to get rid of him.

Deeper meanings?

The story is gripping and totally convincing despite the nightmarish strangeness of the basic idea. If you are still following my medical analogy, it would seem that the patient's family are totally lacking in empathy for him. Could this happen to a patient with a stroke? At first the idea seems unacceptable. But I think that together with pity and concern when we are confronted with someone who is suddenly transformed and distorted by illness, we may also have to struggle with feelings of fear, irritation, anger and disgust. Why has this person done this to himself? How can he expect me to understand his bizarre speech? Why doesn't he walk properly? Why does he make such a mess for me to clear up? Can't he try harder? But that's just one way of reading the story. On another level, as I have already suggested, it is worth remembering that in Franz Kafka's own home in Prague (not unlike the flat where the Samsa family live) he felt crushed and bullied by his father, who seemed to treat him like a worthless insect. So what is The Metamorphosis 'really' about? Is it a piece of disguised autobiography, a metaphor of sickness, a plea for inter-racial (or inter-species) tolerance – or just a story about a man who became a beetle? Possibly all of the above and more besides. Certainly no one who reads this story will ever forget it.

The Burrow (1923)

Here we have another of Kafka's greatest animal stories. This time there is no transformation from the human, but the story is told in the first person so it's clear that Kafka, the author, identifies closely with his unnamed animal hero. But what kind of animal is he? In the first sentence he tells us proudly that he has completed the construction of his burrow so he is obviously some sort of furry animal that makes its home underground. He is very nervous and vulnerable: but he is also carnivorous so he can't be a rabbit. I think he must be a mole or possibly a badger. This is Kafka's version of *The Wind in the Willows*.

Like the Mole and the Badger, this animal lives in a hole in the ground of which he is very proud. But the main purpose of the burrow is to provide our little friend with a place of safety. How can its existence be kept secret from other animals in the forest? 'All that can be seen from the outside is a big hole.' But this is merely a false entrance whose purpose is to deceive any nosy strangers. The real entrance is a thousand paces away, covered with a movable layer of moss. Why is there no solid protective door? Because our friend might have to escape in a hurry at any moment. Even when he is lying snugly in the depths of his secret home, he is tortured by fears of the intrusion of some long-snouted creature who might blunder in to rob or kill him. He draws some comfort from the thought that he might be able to overcome and eat the robber himself if it wasn't too big. But he is conscious of losing his youthful strength – and, in his mind at least, he has many enemies. As he tells us:

> ... it's not only by external enemies that I am threatened. There are also enemies in the bowels of the earth. I have never seen them, but legend tells of them and I firmly believe in them. They are creatures of the inner earth; not even legend can describe them. Their very victims can scarcely have seen them; they come, you hear the scratching of

*their claws just under your ground which is their element, and already
you are lost.*

Are you ready with a diagnosis? Yes, this poor little creature who
has confided in us so eagerly, is depressed, paranoid, subject to
anxiety attacks and is more than a touch obsessional. But you
can't help being fond of him, and very much concerned for his
safety as well as his mental health. Do we ever feel threatened
like he does? You bet we do. It might be the fear of walking into
a terrorist attack or just the uneasy feeling that someone or something is out to get us. And, as our patients tell us every day, the
danger is just as likely to come from within.

A tour of the burrow

All the same, this burrow looks safe enough. Our furry friend
now takes us on a conducted tour of his home. He lives there alone
and seems to prefer it that way. The most beautiful thing about
the burrow, he tells us, is the stillness. As we go deeper in we see
that it is amazingly large. The passages seem to go on for hundreds
of yards and every so often they are widened to form a cosy little
round chamber. In these he can curl up happily, warm and snug.
Yes, it is a bit womb-like, isn't it? Now we are nearly in the centre
of the complex where all the tunnels converge on a huge chamber.
This is the Castle Keep, a much larger cave in which our friend
keeps his food stores. These would appear to consist of the
carcases of smaller animals he has killed and dragged down to
dine on at his leisure. The place is full of powerful smells but he
isn't a vegetarian and to him the odours are delicious. It's like
living in a gourmet restaurant. And yet, the painful thing is that
although he has this extensive and beautiful underground mansion,
which he has built entirely himself, he is constantly afraid that
someone or something is going to break in and spoil it all. His
thoughts constantly return to defensive precautions. Perhaps
more food should be stored in other chambers in case the Castle
Keep is captured? Or would the presence of food in other rooms
give away his presence to a casual intruder? The poor animal
can't decide and he keeps changing his mind.

Watching from outside

Every so often, he tells us, he leaves the burrow for a while so that he can observe it from the outside. First of all he works his way through the complicated labyrinth of passages near the opening. This he has created to make it harder for any strange animal to find its way to the heart of the burrow, even if it discovers the entrance. When he reaches the mossy cushion that blocks his front door he rests underneath it for a while, wondering if it might not be more sensible to stay inside: for suppose something sees him emerging and his secret is betrayed? But no, he has to go and inspect the outside world for signs of danger. Once outside he can do a bit of hunting to replenish his larder. But soon he is drawn back to the concealed entrance of the burrow: he finds a good hiding place and keeps watch on his own front door – for days and nights – to see if any other animal has discovered it. It is actually very reassuring to see the occasional animal going to and fro, oblivious of the burrow's existence. Strangely, at these times, he feels more secure outside the burrow than inside it! Lying there, on watch, he ruminates anxiously about his situation. He would love to go down again – but suppose some small creature follows him and gives the game away? Or it might be one of his own kind who would want to take over his lovely home. This thought fills him with rage, and he imagines how he would kill the enemy, drag his body into the burrow and add it to his food stores. Perhaps it would be better to find a friend to confide in: someone who would agree to watch outside while he was snug in the burrow. But no, that's out of the question, who could you trust?

At last he plucks up courage and dives down again into his home, trembling with fear in case he has been spotted. All appears to be well and he is temporarily reassured. He happily begins a routine inspection of the burrow: checking all the rooms and passages for minor damage. Then, exhausted, he falls asleep.

What's making that noise?

When he wakes, he becomes aware of a new source of worry: 'an almost inaudible whistling noise'. What can it be and where is it coming from? Perhaps it was caused by some of the harmless 'small fry' who also inhabit the burrow. They may have been doing a bit of minor tunnelling and created some peculiar air currents where their tiny passages intersect with his big ones. The best thing would be to find out exactly where the noise is coming from and either get rid of it or forget about it. But although he listens and searches, calmly at first and then with increasing dismay, he can't find the source. Now I don't know if you have ever been bothered by strange noises in hotel bedrooms or even in your own home, but I certainly have. I have been known to pester receptionists demanding a change of room in the middle of the night and there have been occasions (my wife will confirm this) when the mysterious sounds of the domestic central heating pump have nearly driven me crazy. So I have some idea what the poor old burrowing animal is going through. I regard his plight with compassion and empathy. Maybe you think it is all a delusion, but if so, you will have to section me as well.

The great beast

So what is to be done? The noise seems to be transmitted through all the walls of the burrow: only in the centre of the Castle Keep is it entirely absent. Sometimes, teasingly, it appears to stop, only to start up again (just like my central heating). The burrower becomes convinced that something is tunnelling towards him. He considers digging a wide trench in the direction of the noise and going on grimly until he finds the cause. Then he becomes possessed with the thought that it must be a single large animal, 'a great beast', which is tunnelling along furiously and making the ground reverberate for miles around. Perhaps it is digging a burrow of its own, unaware of the closeness of its neighbour's desirable residence. Perhaps it will change direction and disappear, minding its own business. But no, it seems more likely that before long, the great beast will break into his own burrow and there will be a horrible confrontation in which 'we shall both blindly bare our teeth and claws'. If only the beast would alter its plan slightly and change the course of its tunnelling; maybe they could co-exist. No, that would be impossible …

At about this point the narrative breaks off. The burrower's story may have been left unfinished. According to one source, the last few pages were destroyed by Kafka's girl friend, Dora, who cared for him lovingly in his last illness. *The Burrow* was one of the last stories he wrote before he succumbed to tuberculosis of the chest and larynx. Perhaps the whistling of the beast was the wheezing in his bronchial passages as the tuberculous process tunnelled steadily towards him.

In fact, the story doesn't need a tidy ending. Like the burrow, it is carefully and beautifully constructed and I think it's perfect just the way it is. Although it's obsessional and paranoid it's often very funny as well. As with the beetle in *The Metamorphosis*, Kafka disguises himself as an animal in order to share some of his deepest feelings with us – quite a privilege. And the next time a patient comes to tell you that the strange knocking noises in the walls of his flat are being made deliberately by the neighbours, who are out to get him, you might remember the burrower and write him a really good Housing Letter.

Josephine the Singer, or The Mouse Folk (1924)

This is a beautiful, relatively little-known Kafka story. I find it incredibly moving – even if it is about mice. Why mice? Well, as with everything by Kafka, there are all sorts of interpretations to be made and inner meanings to be discovered, but we'll come to those later. The story begins: 'Our singer is called Josephine. Anyone who has not heard her does not know the power of song.' The speaker is a member of the 'mouse people' (OK, he's a mouse) and he seems to be telling us that his community is fortunate enough to have a mouse singer who is not only musically gifted but also amazingly charismatic. Nothing less than a superstar. One thinks of Judy Garland or Edith Piaf or perhaps Maria Callas. And of course, like these legendary human divas, Josephine is not only wonderful but also self-absorbed, volatile, manipulative – and vulnerable.

As with human superstars, there are many unanswered questions and paradoxes surrounding Josephine. Many mice adore her but others try to be more aloof and critical. Our mouse narrator gives us the facts and tries to explain the phenomenon.

The first problem, he tells us, is that the mouse people are 'quite unmusical'. Perhaps Josephine is so good that even unmusical mice are moved, just as non-opera lovers will respond to Pavarotti. No, that can't be the explanation because actually her singing is 'nothing out of the ordinary'. Worse than that, it may not even be singing at all but something our friend describes as 'piping' (or in German, 'pfeiffen'). It seems that piping is something that all mice do effortlessly. It's not so much an art as 'an expression of our life'. I sometimes wonder if Kafka is really talking about 'squeaking', which is what real mice do: but piping seems to be a more accurate translation. More devastatingly, he goes on to say that Josephine's piping is no better than anyone else's. Maybe not even average! So why does she have so much influence over the life of the community?

Well, for one thing, to appreciate her effect, you have to *be* there, watching a live performance. Josephine is the only mouse who makes a ceremonial performance out of piping – that's partly what makes her special. And if anyone ever suggests that any mouse can pipe and most of them do, or tries to mention her art and ordinary piping in the same breath, she can get very sarcastic and unpleasant.

The narrator goes on to tell us that life for the mouse people is full of anxiety. 'Every day brings surprises, apprehensions, hopes and terrors.' It is when things get particularly bad for the people that Josephine comes into her own. 'There she stands, the delicate creature, shaken by vibrations, especially below the breast bone, so that one feels anxious for her.' She may decide to sing almost anywhere: at once, the news flies round and the mice gather about her, 'warmly pressed body to body', under her spell and drawing strength from her performance. But she is temperamental, and like all charismatic singers she needs her public as much as they need her. If the crowd doesn't gather quickly enough 'she stamps her feet, swearing in most unmaidenly fashion; she actually bites'. I find the idea of the great singer getting so furious that she bites people very funny – I can imagine Maria Callas biting someone, backstage at La Scala.

But none of the mouse people would ever laugh at Josephine. She is 'this frail creature, needing protection' and they treat her as a national treasure. Josephine, on the other hand, believes that it is she who protects the people by her singing whenever the news is bad or danger threatens (as all too frequently it does). If her singing 'does not drive away the evil, at least it gives us the strength to bear it'.

The tragic life of the mouse people

Kafka (in his guise as mouse commentator) then goes on to tell us more about the life of the community. Among the mouse people, he says, 'there is no age of youth, scarcely the briefest childhood'. Life is so precarious that the little ones must grow up very quickly and be able to take care of themselves. On the other hand the mouse people are very fertile: 'hardly does a child appear than it is no more a child while behind it new childish faces are already crowding so fast and so thick that they are indistinguishable, rosy with happiness'. This may seem a bit alarming if you are thinking 'rodent pests': but Kafka's words seem to evoke tragic, human children, denied a proper childhood, a situation which we have seen described in our newspapers only too often.

As if to compensate for their lost childhood, the adult mice remain rather childish and frivolous (although they also have plenty of common sense). And yet, says Kafka, they are also prematurely old, subject to feelings of weariness and hopelessness. When Josephine is performing:

> in the brief intervals between their struggles, our people dream. ....
> And into these dreams Josephine's piping drops note by note. ...
> Something of our poor brief childhood is in it, something of lost
> happiness that can never be found again, but also something of active
> daily life, of its small gaieties, unaccountable and yet springing up
> and not to be obliterated.

This is all beautifully written (and translated) and I find it very moving. But then I start to think: I'm getting a lump in my throat about *mice?* Is this a Disney film or a Kafka story? Just who are these mouse people? Who is Kafka really talking about? Well, I think that, at one level, he is talking about real talking mice people who have sprung, fully equipped with human emotions, from his fertile imagination. But what are the dangers which threaten them? Mouse traps? Poisoned cheese? Are there lots of cats in Prague? Perhaps. But if we think of the mice as a minority community, disliked and despised, they instantly become the Jews of Prague. Kafka did not live to see the destruction of his community in the Holocaust (he died in 1924), but many people think that in his writings he uncannily predicted it. And his sisters were all killed in the death camps.

So if the mice are the Jewish people (or any persecuted, vulnerable minority) who is Josephine? Again there are many layers. Kafka was very interested in the traditional Yiddish theatre, which flourished in Eastern Europe in his youth. He may have seen and heard a prima donna who piped charismatically like Josephine. But there is another explanation. ...

Let's just finish the story and learn a bit more about the character and aspirations of the famous *chanteuse*. For a long time back, Kafka tells us, Josephine has been fighting for exemption from the need to do an ordinary job to earn her living. In other words, she demands state support so that she can devote herself to her art. She wants respect and official recognition for her gifts and her unique role in the community. But the people won't have it. Although they love and admire Josephine they are deaf to her pleas and insist that she does her day job as well. A little while ago, she threatened to reduce the quality of her singing, 'to cut short her grace notes' if her demands were not met. Unfortunately no one seemed to notice the difference and, after a while, she announced that her grace notes would be restored to their former glory. More recently, she has complained that she is unable to stand and sing because her foot has been injured at work. Her supporters plead with her to sing and eventually she does, but she seems weary and dispirited. The latest Josephine news is that she has vanished completely! But the people bear her absence stoically. In the last paragraph the narrator speculates about her future. He thinks that it can't be long before 'her last notes sound and die into silence'. Will she be a treasured memory? Not really.

'She is a small episode in the eternal history of our people, and the people will get over the loss of her.'

Kafka and Josephine

The story of Josephine was probably the last thing Kafka ever wrote. He was exhausted and dying of tuberculosis of the lungs and larynx, at the age of 41. He was living in his parents' house, being cared for by his devoted Dora, perhaps the only woman with whom he was ever properly in love. So the story can be seen as Kafka's ironic farewell to life, literature and the community in which he had grown up. The 'mouse people' of Prague had tolerated this strange, awkward young man in their midst and even acknowledged his talents to some extent. But they never really took his writing seriously or understood why it was so important to him. They insisted that he continue to work in his office by day and do his writing at night. So he would give instructions for his unpublished work to be burned and very likely he would soon be forgotten: just 'a small episode in the eternal history of our people'. And if you are still not convinced that Kafka saw himself as Josephine, I think you should know that after he had finished the story, he said to his doctor friend Robert Klopstock, in a voice weakened by tuberculosis of the larynx: 'I think I started to investigate squeaking at just the right moment.'

Whether or not you like the idea of Kafka as Josephine (instead of Joseph K, his male alter ego) doesn't really matter. You are free to interpret the story in any way that occurs to you; or, as with the other animal stories, simply take it at face value as a story about mice. It remains a brilliant and final example of Kafka's genius; moving, intriguing, amusing and totally original.

The texts

'The Metamorphosis', 'The Burrow' and 'Josephine the Singer, or The Mouse People' can be found in *The Penguin Complete Short Stories of Franz Kafka* (various translators, edited by Nahum N Glatzer, published by Vintage and subsequently by Penguin, 1983).

More recently (1991) Penguin published the stories in a translation by Malcolm Pasley. They are in two volumes: *Metamorphosis and Other Stories* also contains 'Josephine the Singer'; 'The Burrow' can be found in *The Great Wall of China and Other Short Works.*

Postscript: It's the tale that wags the dog: more on Kafka by Alistair Stead

John Salinsky has chosen to highlight those notable short narratives among Kafka's works which are loosely categorised as 'animal stories', i.e. stories in which animals figure as protagonists or narrators or both. However, given that we are dealing with a notoriously equivocal writer, we might hesitate about our categories. First, are these all 'stories'? Many short – often extremely short – pieces by Kafka (whether they feature animals or not) are minimally narrative, more like meditations on a theme, where a trace of an anecdote or the occasional event punctuates some exposition of a situation or reflection on an idea. They sometimes read like mini-essays or concentrated, puzzling perversions of accepted wisdom. See *The Tower of Babel*, or *Prometheus*, or *The Spring*.

The *Metamorphosis* is most obviously a long short story with recognisable human agents, a simple plot and powerful closure, but *The Burrow* may be deemed to begin to depart from such a model as we attend to a rather attenuated tale encompassing a limited number of events. The accent seems to be on the futile circuits of the paranoid monologue of the first-person narrator. The sense that this monologue could go on forever may reflect the contention among many scholars that many of Kafka's works, particularly the later ones, remain unfinished, are only fragments, or have, to Kafka's exacting mind, unsatisfactory conclusions. (He considered, after all, that he had botched the ending of Gregor Samsa's transformation!) This seems more likely in the case of a late work which I would like to add, in a moment, to John's impressive selection: *Investigations of a Dog*. Although *Josephine the Singer* traces the doomed trajectory of its central figure in a pattern reminiscent of *The Metamorphosis*, but with a gentler irony, the narrative is propelled not so much by distinctive happenings as by the anxious rumination on the significance of the nature and fate of Josephine as some token of the curious relationship of the individual to the group. The narrator, not Kafka, appears to be some kind of speculative historian of the 'mouse folk' (the subtitle).

Even if we stick with our crude definition of 'animal stories', such works have been, quite plausibly, perceived and discussed as something else, as 'artist stories'. This can be most persuasively argued in the case of the diva Josephine, where it is only in that subtitle to her story that she and her kind are referred to as mice. The unidentified narrator of *The Burrow*, obsessed with the design and construction of his defensive home, may be considered a kind of architect. (Philip Roth, a great Kafka fan, sees a portrait of the artist in there.) Among the many kinds of interpretation wished upon what is commonly agreed to be the greatest of Kafka's tales, the approach through the figure of the artist may appear less rewarding than several others: the transformed Gregor is only very loosely analogous to the lonely, tortured writer of the modern tradition. John writes of how Kafka 'disguises himself as an animal in order to share some of his deepest feelings with us', and those feelings may often include his serious doubts about his vocation as an artist or the value of art at all, but just as often draw upon the sometimes quite distinct torments of the mind and body of Franz, son, lover, friend, clerk, citizen, Jew. If we accept the form of the insect-like creature as such a disguise, then we may be struck by the fact that the protagonist is, or has been until now, a rather commonplace, hard-working commercial traveller (the routine business side of Kafka if you will) with a strictly limited aesthetic sense. If he is so attached, even in his terribly transfigured state, to that framed magazine picture of a lady in furs it seems likely that we have one of the author's grim little jokes, for the picture is not only a genteel-seeming pin-up rather than a masterpiece of painting, but also a subtler erotic fetish, most probably alluding to the sado-masochism of Leopold Sacher-Masoch's infamous novel, *Venus in Furs*, whose title points to the dominatrix adored by this masochist protagonist with pretensions to being a self-sacrificing hero. The art of music figures more strikingly in the Samsa story and John's account touches on that potentially pivotal moment when Gregor responds to the appeal of his sister's performance on the violin: 'Was he an animal that music had such an effect on him?' Is this a sympathetic rendering of Gregor's residual human nature, manifested in this unique aesthetic responsiveness? Vladimir Nabokov for one, though a great admirer of the tale, reads it differently, regarding Gregor's deluded estimation of his sister's pitiful performance on the violin as evidence that the brother succumbs like an animal to the primitive emotional appeal of the sounds and indulges himself with another self-sacrificial fantasy in planning to fund a proper musical training for her – a reading which would find some support from equivocations in other stories about musical art (*Josephine* and *Investigations*) and ambivalence registered in Kafka's *Diaries*. Such dissenting readings are not intended to be dogmatic reinterpretations, but merely serve to underline the difficulties with which these ever-elusive stories, replete with contradictions, present us once we seek to pin down any comparatively simple meaning.

Initially, one tends to think that imagining (or disguising) one's self as an animal in literature is an invitation for the reader to empathise. The old schoolroom exercise 'A Day in the Life of a Dog' usually proves an irresistible opportunity for cross-species identification. And we may ask whether we are to be uncritically fond of Gregor or Josephine, or, more provocatively, of the badger or mole who seems to narrate in his own person *The Burrow*. What customarily occurs in the Kafka piece, I would maintain, is that the writer supplies distancing devices to cool or complicate any over-eager identifications. It is surely worthy of note that the chief figures in the tales discussed by John are all vermin; the word for vermin, *ein Ungeziefer*, is used notably to describe Gregor when he awakens to his transformation. 'Vermin' may refer not only to obnoxious insects, but also to troublesome animals such as mice or creatures who destroy game; badgers and moles have their human enemies, too! (Compare the seductively canny narrator of 'The Stowaway', the first chapter of Julian Barnes' vermiculate *A History of the World in 10½ Chapters*, who winningly mocks the orthodox Judeo-Christian reading of the story of Noah's Ark but is eventually revealed to be the devious and destructive woodworm.) Other impressive creatures in Kafka's bestiary are either healthy predators like the panther and the jackals, or appear worryingly out of place, like 'The Animal in the Synagogue' or 'The Leopard in the Temple'. It will be objected that some of these beasts, like Barnes' woodworm, have been sympathetically and humorously presented (mice are often cute, as in the recent *Stuart Little*, and as the targets of cats – the off-stage enemy in the wars reported in *Josephine*? – they may easily be associated with the persecuted Jews). Nevertheless, a doubt is planted in our mind. One critic goes so far as to state bluntly that Gregor is, literally and metaphorically, a louse, which gets one thinking about the degree to which he can be held responsible in some sense for what goes on. Josephine, the squeaky mouse, is no great shakes as a singer, throws tantrums, manipulates her audience, then fades away, and may eventually, without much fuss, be forgotten even by her own kind. That garrulous burrowing creature creates his own problem (making a mountain out of a molehill?) and is more aggressive than at first appears. Always there are counter-indications of this sort in the spirit of the author's addiction to the shockingly paradoxical. Take Kafka's dog (or dogs). He never turns up as faithful companion, man's best friend. Kafka's most famous book, *The Trial*, ends memorably with the terrible death of Josef K at the hands of two killers. The last words represent K's final vision of things: '"Like a dog!" he said: it was as if he meant the shame of it to outlive him.'

In the *Diaries*, comparisons with dogs are not flattering, overshadowed as they are perhaps both by some common usage ('son of a bitch'), the etymology of 'cynic' (dog-like), and by Kafka's father's vicious dismissal of his son's friendship with the actor Löwy with the proverb: 'Whoever lies down with dogs gets up with fleas.' So when in *Investigations*, the narrator presents himself as a dog, for all the charming naïvety and seductive candour of the exposition, suspicions may arise that a more mixed quality is on display.

In a rambling retrospect, an old dog claims to be engaged in scientific research, portraying himself as partly alienated from his kind by such intellectual ambition but devoted all the same to his 'dog-nation' and totally convinced that all answers reside in dogs: 'For what else is there apart from dogs?' An early experience of coming across seven dogs dancing on their hind legs in a lighted space to some wondrous music proves decisive in exciting his curiosity, directed at first at the question of how dogs obtain their food and, later, more briefly, at the mystery of the 'music' they make to procure such food. His work is frustrated by the silence of his fellow dogs and by the failure of his personal experiment in fasting (to test whether food would turn up without the ritual either of scratching and watering of the ground or of looking up and leaping into the air to catch it).

Inspired to return to the mystery of the dogs' music by the impression he has received that a strange hunting dog has been unconsciously singing to him when he was on the point of dying, he now relies on an instinct stronger than scientific reasoning and the account ends with exultation in the freedom that his instinct brings him. It will be seen from this radically foreshortened summary of an excessively earnest, self-involved and self-contradictory narration that there is a foretaste of Beckettian absurdity in the futile questing and the self-sabotaging line of argument which accompanies it, for the bold claims or aspirations to be a scientific researcher are gradually superseded by confessions of lack of expertise in science in general and in the spheres of nutrition and music in particular. In any case, his researches, as he has aged, have become only intermittent and, to the reader, appear transparently grotesque in method. His apparently rational project then collapses into irrationalism.

The dog tells his story, we gather, when old, enfeebled, inactive, perhaps in some kind of nursing home – or even an asylum? After all, he not only fails to recognise, even retrospectively, that the seven dogs were performing in a circus act and that the puzzle about the origins of the dog's food (and much else) would be resolved if he would acknowledge the canine dependence on the presence and agency of human beings in his world, but he openly admits that in this 'world of lies', even he, who hungers after truth, is born 'a citizen of falsehood'. Thus, first-person narrators in Kafka regularly turn out to be detectably unreliable (and if the story is told in the third person but adhering closely to the consciousness of one character, like Gregor, there's no guarantee that he, no matter how much he suffers, has a truer vision than the others in the story). Like most beast fables (*vide* Barnes' woodworm) the dog story depends on the impossible: animals don't talk, or write, and their motives may be less complicated than our own. Kafka, for his part, forces us to recognise this. The taciturnity of the dogs (they only appear to sing or speak to the narrator) points up the absurdity of the narrator himself, supposedly addressing an audience of dogs, but at a late point admitting that he is, like his fellows, 'silent'. How then can he communicate with *us*?

Which brings us to a central issue: how animal-like are the supposed animals in these pieces? Here Kafka seems to start from the old beast fables (like Aesop's or La Fontaine's), where we encounter short allegories or parables of the human condition in which whatever is said about or by the animals may be translated into a moralised commentary on ourselves, a tradition which finds its outstanding twentieth-century representative in George Orwell's brilliant political satire, *Animal Farm*. Technically, animals are rendered in a cartoon-like way. That doesn't mean Disney-cute: the burrower, for example, uses claws and teeth to defend himself against the menace of his unseen foe. Kafka tends to mix some graphic simplification with subtler shadings, holding back the grotesque material view by having the animal narrate in a parody of human self-justification or philosophical rumination. Thus, the supposedly fertilising watering of the ground in *Investigations* will eventually be decoded as the dog's urination, or the singing of the mice in *Josephine* (that they are mice is vouchsafed only in the subtitle, and Kafka even has his little joke by remarking that Josephine's public are *'mäusschen still '*, 'as quiet as mice') is, by the use of the ambiguous 'piping', not immediately identified as the more realistic 'squeaking'. *The Metamorphosis* is a special case, of course, as Gregor gradually loses his human self to a more and more verminous appearance and destiny – the dustbin. But the ethical issues of the lightly didactic beast fable are complicated in Kafka by more than one feature.

First, there is the more serious post-Darwinian attention he pays to the animality of the human beings portrayed or implied in the narratives. The focus on animals in the fiction naturally brings to the fore the evolutionary themes of the survival of the fittest, of mutation and adaptation, of the relation of the individual to the species, and these themes may be perceived to translate readily into human contexts. They resonate in aesthetic, religious and ethnic spheres, whether we are invited to assess the (usually doomed) strategies adopted by the isolated artist or thinker to survive in a hostile environment, a philistine culture, or we wish to extrapolate from these tricky allegories ironic reflections on a beleaguered Jewish identity (a stronger tendency among latter-day critics), whether this invokes tensions between Jews and Gentiles, secularism and orthodox belief, or the assimilationist and Zionist tendencies to which Kafka gave allegiance at different times in his life. Only half playfully, for he regularly employs and enjoys puns. The writer draws attention, through plays on his surname, to his kinship with animal life: Kafka (*kavka* in Czech) means jackdaw, with whom he explicitly identifies himself in a letter. In another story and his *Diaries*, he evokes the Hunter Gracchus, born of a dream-double, where the strange name Gracchus in all likelihood alludes to *graculus*, Latin for jackdaw. When Roth examines the most frequently published photograph of his hero, he sees 'a burrower's face'.

More obviously significant is the ambiguity in the presentation of the ape who gives *A Report for an Academy*. His circus performance as a human may be patronised as amusing caricature or seen as a deliberately satirical reminder of our common ancestry. It is significant that animal and artist stories converge often enough when the animal is a performer, like the seven dogs and Josephine. Kafka himself was no great singer or dancer, by all accounts, but he loved to read out loud the stories he admired, turning them into dramatic performances. Then, the author also inserts more naturalistic touches into what might conceivably be read as fairy-tale and folk-tale creatures, bringing them into disturbing proximity to the world of our common experience. Thus Nabokov expends much energy on trying to identify what variety of beetle Gregor might have become, tantalised by the supply of just enough plausible detail for the keen lepidopterist to believe he is on the scent of a definite classification. But he has to admit an exemplary defeat: 'neither Gregor nor Kafka saw that beetle any too clearly'. And, in the end, the same goes for all the wee beasties. For Kafka deals not only in hybrid stories (mixtures of fairy tale, Gothic horror, Yiddish family drama and cool realism), but in stories of hybrids, creatures that seem to be in transition, crossing the boundaries between kinds. The 'monstrous' creatures are there, first and foremost, to tell a tale of indefinite import.

To take a final instance: in *Investigations of a Dog*, it has been argued that Kafka is rebelling against the Zionism he had been drawn to by satirising a Zionist narrator in his dog researcher who has contempt for the 'dog's life' led by the Jews wandering in the Diaspora, and is obsessed with dietary restrictions and adherence to ritual. When the narrator hears of 'air dogs' (very small, fancy dogs who seem to hover in the air), he comically fails, of course, to realise that they are lap dogs, but the term in German *'Lufthunde'* seems to be a play on the Yiddish *'Luftmensch'* (those who have to depend on the community for support; idle or impractical folk), which can be interpreted, in the Zionist reading, as mystical Jews. To compare the Jews to dogs at all is a manifestly risky business, of course, and we may still hear Antonio's affront to Shylock, 'cut-throat dog'. It may be argued, however, that Kafka is more interested in an internecine struggle *within* Judaism. Still, faced with Kafka's wide-ranging deployment of enigmatic animal characters in the service of intellectually provocative but often moving and humorous meditations or narratives, we should perhaps rise to the challenge of appreciating the painful and eloquent diversity of the new tricks that this (prematurely) old dog has got up to.

Further reading

Investigations of a Dog is to be found in *The Great Wall of China and Other Short Works* (Penguin, 1991). *The Diaries of Franz Kafka 1910–23* were edited by Max Brod (Penguin, 1964). Vladimir Nabokov on *The Metamorphosis* appears in his *Lectures on Literature* (Weidenfeld and Nicolson, 1980) and Philip Roth's 'I Always Wanted You to Admire My Fasting; or, Looking at Kafka' in his *Reading Myself and Others* (Cape, 1975). Extract from *The Trial* by Franz Kafka and translators Willa and Edwin Muir published by Secker and Warburg. Used by permission of The Random House Group Limited.

12

Women in Love

by DH Lawrence (1920)

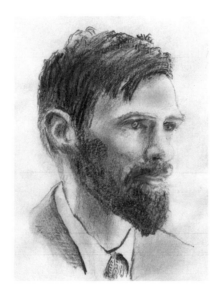

A difficult book – a difficult writer?

Most of the books I have chosen to write about in *Medicine and Literature* have been old favourites that have pushed themselves eagerly forward for consideration. This time I have decided to take another look at an author whom I have always found heavy going in the past. When I was growing up there were always plenty of Penguin novels by DH Lawrence lying around for me to dip into: my medical student elder brothers seemed to be reading them when they needed a change from *Gray's Anatomy*.

I got on quite well with Lawrence's early success, *Sons and Lovers*, although I was puzzled and frustrated by Paul Morel's failure to marry his girlfriend, Miriam. But when I tried some of the later novels I was disconcerted and confused by Lawrence's wild and wonderful idiosyncratic prose style. He would begin with a bit of straightforward narrative and then suddenly take off into what seemed to be a very mannered and overwrought language which I couldn't follow and in which I lost my grasp on the characters and the plot.

By 1960, when *Lady Chatterley's Lover* was finally published in Britain, I was a student. My friends and I all queued up to get hold of this notorious sexy book, which had emerged triumphantly from its criminal trial at the Old Bailey. A few years later (1969) Lawrence was in the news again with the appearance of Ken Russell's film version of *Women in Love*. If you are old enough, you may remember the scene in which Alan Bates and Oliver Reed wrestled naked in front of the fire. My copy of the book has Alan Bates and Jenny Linden on the cover just about to kiss. I must have bought it after I saw the film, but I don't think I ever finished it. The time for Lawrence and me to wrestle together in the library had not yet arrived.

Now, over 30 years later, we have finally got to grips and it's very exciting. It started when I was having a bit of a clear out of the shelves, came across my old copy of *Women in Love* and started reading it again. This time, I found the writing in some of the chapters quite astonishing. Reading them was like listening to a symphony orchestra in full flood. Wagner and Debussy were the composers who mainly came to my inner ear. But you can't read a book for the music alone. What about the story and the characters? I could just about follow the plot but I could not get the hang of the furious arguments about life, love, art, death, dissolution and personal freedom, which were constantly breaking out. My brows furrowed in perplexity but I didn't give up. I knew that I needed to find out more about Lawrence's life and how he came to create this strangely beautiful fictional world.

The life of David Herbert Lawrence

He was born in Eastwood, Nottingham, in 1885. His father was a coal miner but his mother was a bit more middle class and a lot more educated. Bert (as he was called) was a bright boy who won a scholarship to Nottingham High School and went on to university. He loved his mother very much and felt that she dominated his life, making it difficult for him to break away. He had plenty of girlfriends as a young man, but found sex problematic and commitment even more difficult. Then he met Frieda, a young German woman, with whom he fell instantly in love. She quickly divorced her husband and they embarked on a passionate marriage, devoted to each other (despite her numerous affairs) but constantly quarrelling. She was his inspiration and she gave him lots of help and encouragement with his work.

Lawrence wrote brilliant poetry, excellent short stories and novels of uneven quality, some much better than others. In creating his characters and stories he drew heavily on his own early years (*Sons and Lovers*) and his relationship with Frieda, who can be found inhabiting most of his principal heroines. He used caricatures of his friends to fill minor roles in his novels, giving rise to a good deal of pain and resentment. He was also very much occupied with working out his own philosophical ideas, and was influenced by a number of thinkers, including Nietszche and some obscure medieval theologians. His friend Bertrand Russell was one of those who thought that Lawrence's ideas came perilously close to fascism, although he was never active in politics. He could be racist and anti-Semitic (although some of his best friends were Jewish). He believed that men should always be superior to women and that romantic love deprived people of freedom. He was the high priest of sex but he wasn't very good at it; he believed that marriage was for life and, although he was loved by many women, he stayed faithful to Frieda. The Lawrences spent much of their life travelling in Europe and America and found it difficult to settle anywhere. His books were controversial (mainly because of their sexual frankness) and difficult to publish. *The Rainbow* and *Lady Chatterley's Lover* were both the subjects of criminal trials. Despite his strange ideas, Lawrence impressed everyone who met him with his sheer enjoyment of life and nature. He was fun to be with. Unfortunately his health was always quite frail and he died of tuberculosis in 1930, at the age of 44.

Once I had learned a bit about Lawrence and his relationships with women, I found *Women in Love* much easier to get hold of. In my biographical researches I also learned about the strange beginnings of the book. During the First World War (which he found very disturbing) Lawrence was working on a project provisionally called *The Sisters*. The first part of this eventually became *The Rainbow*, a saga of several generations of the Brangwen family, who live in Lawrence's native Nottinghamshire. *Women in Love* finally emerged as the second part and was not published until 1921. You don't have to read *The Rainbow* first because *Women in Love* is complete in itself and you don't need the back story. But you will enjoy reading it afterwards.

Women in love: the two sisters

Women in Love starts with a conversation between Ursula Brangwen (aged 26) and her younger sister Gudrun (25). Ursula is a schoolteacher and Gudrun is an artist, just returned from a stay in London. Gudrun is the more striking of the two. She is very pretty and wears stylish, colourful clothes. She is lively and amusing, but there is something brittle about her and she is not as confident as she seems. Her sister's pet name for her is 'prune'. Does that mean she is shiny on the surface but dried up inside?

The girls are talking about marriage, much as sisters might do in a nineteenth-century novel such as *Middlemarch*. But the time is about 1912 and the big difference is that these sisters don't see marriage as inevitable or necessarily desirable. The prospect of any man one knows coming home every evening and giving one a kiss is 'impossible'. They definitely don't want babies either, thank you very much. So what do the girls want? Gudrun talks bravely about taking a big jump: ' "If one jumps over the edge one is bound to land somewhere". "But isn't it very risky?" asked Ursula.'

So instead of jumping over the edge, they walk out of their parents' house and into Beldover, which is a small colliery town in the Midlands, rather like Lawrence's native Eastwood. Both girls are repelled by the dirt and the poverty of the mean streets (although Gudrun finds the grimy masculinity of the colliers exciting). They emerge, with relief, into the country and reach the prosperous village of Willey Green. It's a spring day and the flowers are coming out. The village church is preparing for a posh wedding: one of the daughters of Mr Crich the local mine owner is about to get hitched, and Ursula and Gudrun, after their conversation on the subject, are intensely curious. From a suitably screened vantage point they watch the principals arriving; and Lawrence takes the opportunity of introducing us to the two young men with whom the sisters are going to fall in love. First to appear is Gerald Crich, the mine owner's eldest son, who makes an immediate impression on Gudrun. 'There was something northern about him which magnetised her. In his clear northern flesh and his fair hair was a glisten like sunshine refracted through crystals of ice …. Perhaps he was thirty years old, perhaps more. His gleaming beauty, maleness, like a young good-humoured, smiling wolf, did not blind her to the significant, sinister stillness in his bearing.' We are starting to get some typical Lawrentian descriptive writing now. No wonder Gudrun is fascinated: 'A strange transport took possession of her, all her veins were in a paroxysm of violent sensation … "I shall know more of that man" ', she says to herself. And later: ' "Am I *really* singled out for him in some way, is there really some pale gold arctic light that envelops only us two?" '

Introducing Hermione

Do you find this style of writing a bit over the top? The best thing is not to analyse it too much: just relax and enjoy the sensations as they flood over you. The lyrical strain in Lawrence's writing always swells up like an orchestral crescendo whenever he describes intense feelings. His style targets your sensory receptors and all those emotion-mediating bits of the brain that the neurobiologists are always telling us about.

Now who is this approaching the church? She's a tall, impressive young woman with a long face and a yellow hat with feathers. Let me introduce you to Hermione Roddice, into whose tortured mind we are about to enter. Hermione is the daughter of a baronet and she is 'a new woman, full of intellectuality'. Lawrence modelled her appearance and her low sing-song voice on Lady Ottoline Morrell, who was a fashionable hostess and artistic patron of the time. In character she was actually not a bit like Hermione; she never had an affair with Lawrence, and she was always good to him. So it was very cruel of him to caricature her in this way and she was justifiably upset. Hermione in the book is the current, shortly to be ex-, girlfriend of our chief hero, Rupert Birkin, with whom Ursula is going to have a passionate and tormented relationship. There is a slight problem about whether we call him Rupert or Birkin. The other characters call him Rupert but the narrator (who must be Lawrence) refers to him as 'Birkin', so for the most part I shall do the same. Unlike the strong, healthy, blonde Gerald, Birkin is a thin, pale, intense, rather weedy young man, much like Lawrence himself. We shall find that Lawrence uses Birkin to voice a lot of his disturbing ideas about love and marriage and the purpose of life. Some of his conversations with Ursula echo the furious quarrels he used to have with his wife, Frieda. However, we mustn't make the mistake of thinking that Rupert Birkin *is* Lawrence and that *Women in Love* is just a fictionalised way of delivering the author's philosophical messages. Lawrence himself said: 'Never trust the artist. Trust the tale.' So let's get back to the tale.

Hermione, as she walks to the church, is agonising about Birkin. In spite of her gifts and accomplishments, she feels insecure and incomplete without him. They have been lovers for years, but now he seems determined to break away from her. What do our two sisters think of Birkin? Ursula has spoken to him once or twice, and she wants to know him more. Gudrun says he's attractive, although not to be trusted. But Ursula is already hooked. The wedding goes ahead. The two young men come out of the church, and the girls leave their observation post to go home. We know who is going to be in love with whom. Both the boys are intriguing in their different ways. And the girls? A lot has happened to them since that sceptical conversation about marriage. It's a great opening chapter, and not at all difficult to read.

Birkin and Gerald: men in love?

Chapter 2 takes us to Shortlands, the Crich family home, where we are allowed to attend the wedding party. We meet Mrs Crich, an unhappy, withdrawn mother, who seems to have difficulty in telling her children apart. Except for Gerald, who is her favourite, 'the most wanting of all'. '"I should like him to have a friend,"' his mother tells Birkin, '"he has never had a friend."' And Birkin remembers that, as a boy, Gerald accidentally killed his brother when they were playing with a gun. Will Birkin be the friend that Gerald has always needed? They have a discussion about whether people should be spontaneous, free to act however they like. Gerald, the controlled one, thinks this would be dangerous and would lead to 'everybody cutting everybody else's throat in five minutes.' 'It's a nasty view of things, Gerald,' said Birkin, 'and no wonder you are afraid of yourself and your own unhappiness.' Gerald thinks he talks a lot of nonsense and they seem to be about to have a row. Then there is a pause and the voice of the narrator comes in to tell us that 'There was a strange enmity between the two men, that was very near to love.' Later on in this final paragraph Lawrence says: 'They parted with apparent unconcern, as if their going apart were a trivial occurrence .... Yet the heart of each burned for the other.' Does this mean that Gerald and Birkin are going to become gay lovers? Not quite. But Lawrence believed strongly in the need for a strong and passionate friendship between men, which seems to have a physical and sensual element. We'll come back to the Gerald–Birkin connection a little later. But first I'd like to follow up the two developing boy–girl relationships, starting with Ursula and Birkin.

Sex education with catkins

In Chapter 3 ('Classroom'), Rupert Birkin, who is a school inspector, pays a visit to Ursula's nature class. As it is spring, they are doing hazel catkins. Birkin is most insistent that the children are shown the spiky little red female flowers as well as the long, dangling, yellow male ones. Then Hermione barges in, on Birkin's trail, and she is shown the catkins too. Birkin asks if she has noticed the red female seed-producing flowers and if she knows about pollination. He seems to be asking her if she knows about sex. Hermione protests that the children might be better off just seeing the plant as a whole without 'all this pulling to pieces, all this knowledge'. They start having an embarrassing argument in which he accuses her of having no true sensual 'animal' feelings but wanting only to talk about them 'in your head'.

'He looked at her in mingled hate and contempt, also in pain because she suffered, and in shame because he knew he tortured her. He had an impulse to kneel and plead for forgiveness. But a bitter red anger burned up to fury in him.' And so the tirade goes on. 'How can you have knowledge not in your head?' asks Ursula innocently. 'In the blood', is Birkin's answer. 'When the known world is drowned in darkness – everything must go – there must be the deluge. Then you find yourself in a palpable body of darkness, a demon –.' And he goes on to tell Hermione: 'You are the real devil who won't let life exist.'

What are we to make of this terrible, confusing scene? First of all we are almost certainly witnessing a replay of one of the Lawrence–Frieda husband and wife arguments. We are getting our first dose (through Birkin) of Lawrence's ideas about sex and sensuality – and of course love. The message changes and develops during his lifetime, but there is always an emphasis on 'the blood', which stands for the instinctual and sensual life as against the more calculating operations of the higher brain centres. Meanwhile, Ursula is becoming more aware of her own sensual attraction to Birkin; when he and Hermione leave, she weeps: 'but whether for misery or joy she never knew'.

On the London train

Gerald and Birkin meet again on the train to London, and, as so often happens on trains, they start to confide in each other. Pretty soon Rupert starts expounding his ideas. He thinks that human life in its present form needs to be completely changed. Gerald is the successful manager of his father's colliery business, so naturally he believes life is about work, production and material prosperity. Birkin pours scorn on this misguided attitude but Gerald smiles and doesn't really take his friend's tirade seriously, although he is a bit taken aback when Birkin says he hates him. They start to talk about the aim and object of their lives, the way you do on long train journeys with your best friend whom you hate. And, of course, they talk about love. Birkin declares that he must have love with just one woman for life.

> *'And you mean if there isn't the woman, there's nothing?' said Gerald.*
> *'Pretty well that – seeing there's no God.'*
> *'Then we're hard put to it,' said Gerald. And he turned to look out of the window at the flying golden landscape.*

(I love that turning to look at the flying landscape: only a really great writer would have put that in. Don't ask me why.)

Scene in a Bohemian café

In London the two young men visit a café where all the artists, musicians, writers and fashionable people hang out (Chapter 6, 'Crème de Menthe'). Various real-life members of London Bohemian café society recognised themselves when they read this chapter and some of them sued or never spoke to Lawrence again, but he

didn't care. He wanted to say what he thought about the superficial, pretentious, untrue lives that he saw being lived around
him. There is an attractive girl with a lisp called Pussum, who is
under the protection of one of the artists. Gerald later spends the
night with her (because that's the way he is) but it is only a one-
night stand. Birkin remains aloof. In the morning, when they all
wake up at someone's flat, Gerald notices a primitive Pacific
carving of a pregnant woman. He asks Birkin what he thinks of it
and Birkin tells him that 'it is art' and that it represents 'pure
culture in sensation ... mindless, utterly sensual'. As we read, we
keep getting little lessons about Birkin's Lawrentian creed. This
one reminds us that sensual is good while 'mind' (i.e. too much
intellectualising) is bad. Birkin wants the love of a woman for life
and he is pinning his hopes on Ursula. But will she understand
what love means to a sensual Lawrentian man? We must read on
to find out.

Breadalby

The girls are invited to Hermione's grand country house called
'Breadalby' in the novel and modelled on Lady Ottoline's place at
Garsington. Hermione welcomes them in her affected-sounding
voice. She notes that Gudrun is the more beautiful of the two, but
Ursula is 'more physical, more womanly'. She admires Gudrun's
stockings – as do we all – every day a different colour. Today they
are dark green with black shoes. A walk is proposed, but Birkin
refuses to go and Hermione mocks him by calling him a sulky
little boy. Later they have a really terrible row – along similar lines:
mind versus body. This time Birkin's savage onslaught makes her
feel quite ill. After lunch there is an intellectual conversation
about what the new world order might be like. Poor Hermione
ventures to say that we are all equal in spirit and Birkin turns on
her yet again. He won't accept equality with anyone: 'In the spirit
I am as separate as one star from another.' Later on he feels some
remorse and wanders into her boudoir – only to be violently
bashed on the head with a lapis lazuli paperweight. Hermione at
last gives him a strongly physical message about her feelings. He

is partly stunned but not killed. He stumbles out across the park into the hills, where he takes off all his clothes and rolls in the wet grass, the flowers and the prickly pine needles. He revels in nature's rough but sensual caresses. Clearly it was the right and the only thing to do. We are told that he was ill for several weeks afterwards. But the blow on the head marks the end of Hermione's attachment to Birkin. Will Ursula fare any better?

Gerald and Gudrun

While he is recovering we switch our attention to Gerald. Chapter 9 ('Coal-Dust') is a little virtuoso piece of writing whose purpose is vividly to illustrate something of Gerald's nature. Ursula and Gudrun are waiting at the gate of a railway level crossing when Gerald rides up on his beautiful red Arab mare. The horse is terrified by the noise of the train. Instead of doing the sensible thing, and riding away until it has gone by, he forces the horse to stand with her head at the crossing gate as the train goes past. There is a struggle of wills between man and beast in which Gerald behaves with sickening brutality, driving his spurs into the poor animal's already bleeding flanks. The girls watch in horror and disbelief. As the train passes and the gate finally opens, the horse leaps up past Gudrun who cries out 'in a strange high voice like a gull, or like a witch screaming out from the side of the road: "I should think you're proud."' Something about Gerald's cruel display of masculine superiority and strength seems to have aroused her sexually, I'm sorry to say, and will continue to do so.

Love and marriage, Lawrentian style

The next few chapters focus mainly on Ursula and Birkin. Ursula is by now very attracted to him and wishes he would just say: 'I love you, let's get married', like any normal boy. But that won't happen. She is going to have to listen to him expounding his idiosyncratic philosophy for quite some time and ultimately to decide whether she can reach an accommodation, even if she never completely accepts it. We readers have a similar task ahead of us. But it's all very interesting, and although Lawrence is totally serious he is able to see the ridiculous side of Rupert Birkin's earnest preaching as well. The conversation starts on an island in the lake, continues while they lay carpets in Birkin's new rooms at the old mill and concludes a few days later in a lovely episode illustrated by a cat. The cat will be our reward for listening carefully to all the theory.

So what is Rupert Birkin's take on love and marriage? He begins by saying that humanity is all rotten and the world would be a better place if 'man was swept off the face of the earth'. Then there would be a new creation. Ursula listens and feels a little jealous: she can't help feeling that he would talk in this thrilling way to any girl who listened: and she wants him to care only for *her*. Does he believe in individual love? she asks cautiously. No, he doesn't believe in love at all, it's just an emotion like any other. She wonders how he can be such a priggish Sunday school preacher and at the same time so desirable (in spite of his look of sickness). As for Birkin: 'He looked up at her and saw her face strangely enkindled in her own living fire. Arrested in wonder and in pure, perfect attraction, he moved towards her. She sat like a strange queen, almost supernatural in her glowing smiling richness.'

Could anyone resist a girl like that? I don't think so. Although Rupert continues to preach, telling her that the very word love should be banned, love's old sweet chemistry is working on him even as he speaks. He tells her he is going to give up his job, 'throw everything away, everything – let everything go, to get the very last thing one wants'. Could that be love, Ursula wonders, but Birkin's offer is 'freedom together'.

Is a woman the same as a horse?

They move to Birkin's new rooms at the mill, where they meet up with Gerald and Hermione, who have come to help him move in. Ursula reproves Gerald for his treatment of the horse at the railway crossing. They all discuss whether animals are there simply for the use of humans and should be forced to obey their owners.

Birkin says that a horse has two wills, one to obey its human master and one to be free. ' "And woman is the same as horses," ' he goes on recklessly. ' "With one will she wants to subject herself utterly. With the other she wants to bolt, and pitch her rider to perdition." "Then I'm a bolter," said Ursula, with a burst of laughter.' She has issued her challenge to Birkin: told him what he can expect if he tries to break her like a horse.

When they meet again, Ursula tries to get a clearer understanding of what sort of relationship he wants. It isn't love, it's something 'much more impersonal and harder – and rarer'. You mean you don't love me, says Ursula. Birkin makes it even more difficult by saying he doesn't want Ursula's good looks, her womanly feelings, or her thoughts, opinions or ideas. So what does he want? Oh dear, it's so annoying for a prophet, the way women will harp on love. He tries to explain, but it's difficult to find the words for such a fine, elusive concept. ' "What I want is a strange conjunction with you ... not meeting and mingling ... but an equilibrium, a pure balance of two single beings: – as the stars balance each other." ' Poor Ursula. I think she can see that he is going through a genuine struggle to express his deepest feelings; and that stirs her deeply as well. But his ideas are so strange – and why can't he say he loves her?

Here's the cat

Then comes the cat, Mino, beautifully described as only Lawrence can sketch an animal in words: 'The young cat trotted lordly down the path, waving his tail. He was an ordinary tabby with white paws, a slender young gentleman.' A fluffy female cat seems to be trying to creep past him, 'looking up at him with wild eyes that were green and lovely like great jewels'. I wish I could reproduce the whole cat-mating episode for you but you must read it for yourselves in the chapter called 'Mino'. Meanwhile, here is another choice morsel:

> In a lovely springing leap, like the wind, Mino was upon her, and had boxed her twice, very definitely with a white, delicate fist. She sank

and slid back, unquestioningly. He walked after her, and cuffed her once or twice, leisurely, with sudden little blows of his magic white paws.
'Now why does he do that?' cried Ursula in indignation.
'They are on intimate terms,' said Birkin.

Ursula complains that this is just male bullying. Is this how he wants to treat her? But Birkin argues that Mino is simply trying to bring the fluffy cat into 'a pure stable equilibrium' with him, 'a transcendent and abiding rapport with the single male'. He continues to struggle for the right words to explain how he wants their marriage to be. He comes up with things like: 'a maintaining of the self in mystic balance and integrity – like a star balanced with another star.' 'I don't trust you when you drag in the stars,' she says. 'If you were quite true it wouldn't be necessary to be so far-fetched.' She pleads with him just to call her 'my love'. Finally he kisses her and agrees, 'murmuring in a subtle voice of love, and irony and submission. "I love you then, I'm bored by the rest." "Yes," she murmured, nestling very sweet and close to him.'

So who has won? The parallel with Lawrence and Frieda's real-life marriage suggests that this is merely a truce and that the desperate battle of love and ideology will soon resume.

Love and death on Willey Water

We have now reached Chapter 14, entitled 'Water-party'. This is a long and momentous chapter – almost a little novel by itself. Mr Crich is holding his annual party on the lake for the townsfolk. There are rowing boats and a steamer and a tea tent and picnics. Ursula and Gudrun go along, dressed in all their finery (Gudrun in pink stockings). The two girls go off in a canoe by themselves to a secluded place where Gudrun does a little dance to entertain the Highland cattle. Gerald and Birkin come to find them. Gerald accuses Gudrun of scaring the cattle; she hits him a little blow on the face with the back of her hand (rather like the cat in the previous chapter) and soon they are kissing. Meanwhile Birkin is talking rather gloomily to Ursula about 'the black river of corruption' leading to the end of the world and, perhaps, a new beginning. Darkness falls and lights appear on all the boats. There are some beautiful (and musical) descriptions of the night scene on the water illuminated by colourful paper lanterns. Then there is a tragedy and the mood goes dark and cold. Gerald's little sister Diana falls off the canopy of the launch into the lake. A young doctor dives in after her but neither of them reappears. Gerald plunges into the black water and desperately tries to find them but has to give up.

Ursula and Birkin go to the sluice gate to drain the water out of the lake. Again they talk about the difference between love and the more detached something-beyond-love that Birkin wants to share with Ursula. After a while, sheer physical desire overcomes them and they start to kiss passionately. They may even have sex; it's not entirely clear from the less-than-explicit but very sensual writing. And so, as a new day breaks, our two couples are definitely united in love or, in Birkin's case, the beginnings of something beyond love.

Nevertheless, the tragedy on the lake has depressed and chilled them. Everyone seems to feel tired and ill. Birkin retires to bed exhausted and broods on his relationship with Ursula. He wonders how he can avoid being trapped in 'the hot narrow intimacy between man and wife'. He wants 'to be with Ursula as free as himself, single and clear and cool'. He can't bear 'the merging and clutching, the mingling of love'. To you and me this close entanglement with the one you love may sound entirely satisfactory; but Rupert is a strange, visionary boy and we must be patient with him. So must Ursula. Gerald drops in for a chat and they discuss their love life, the way young men will, except that with Birkin the conversation soon reverts to death and degeneration and how one is to escape from the ordinary to be free and extraordinary. Gerald doesn't really follow the arguments, but both men realise again that they are very attracted to each other. Birkin proposes an oath of blood brotherhood in which they will swear to love each other all their lives. It's not really sexual and yet the way Lawrence describes their feelings for one another is very moving. If you are a straight male reader, have you ever felt like this about another man, quite apart from your love for the woman in your life? You can send me an email. Personally, I believe that it really happens and, when it does, is to be treasured. Gerald feels it too, but he is not keen on swearing the oath, even when Birkin says they can do without the blood-letting. 'We'll leave it till we understand it better,' he says, to his friend's disappointment.

Gerald's father: the old capitalist

To help us to understand Gerald's background better, Lawrence now tells us about his father, Thomas Crich, the industrial magnate. The old man had been a philanthropic employer, always very concerned about the welfare of his miners and their families. Then Gerald grows up and takes over the business with a totally different management style. He introduces modern machinery, cuts costs ruthlessly, and makes everything run very efficiently and profitably. The miners hate him but he doesn't care. Only sometimes he has what we might call panic attacks. Sex with a woman made him feel better for a time; but now 'he felt that his mind needed stimulation before he could be physically aroused'.

Spectacular chapters

Meanwhile, Gudrun is still feeling uncertain about whether being in love with Gerald is a good idea. Whenever she sees him doing something masterful and yes, brutal, she is strongly aroused. In Chapter 18 ('Rabbit') he subdues a very strong pet rabbit, which is struggling to escape from Gudrun's grasp. They both get scratched forearms and feel excited about each other while the rabbit, whose name is 'Bismarck', runs round in circles and then peacefully nibbles some grass. Lawrence always writes brilliantly about animals and this chapter is a classic example.

The next one, Chapter 19, is even better. It's called 'Moony', and for sheer beauty of impressionistic writing it must be the best one in the book. In the late evening, after nightfall, Ursula is wandering by the lake brooding about Birkin, who has been away. She comes to the millpond and is entranced by the reflection of the full moon in the water. Birkin appears on the other side and starts to throw stones, trying to make the moon go away by smashing her reflection.

> *Ursula was aware of the bright moon leaping and swaying, all distorted in her eyes. It seemed to shoot out arms of fire like a cuttlefish. Like a luminous polyp, palpitating strongly before her.... Then again, there was a burst of sound and a burst of brilliant light, the moon had exploded on the water and was flying asunder in flakes of white and dangerous fire.*

That's only a small sample of this dazzling display of writing about light, which goes on for two and a half pages. Nothing else in literature is quite like it: for a comparison you have to think of music by Debussy or a Monet painting. What is young Rupert's quarrel with the moon? She is like the great mother, from whom he is trying to escape. He tries, once again, to explain the kind of relationship he wants to have with Ursula. Still she is doubtful about it and once again they end up kissing.

The next day, we find Rupert brooding over sensual fulfilment. He remembers a wooden African statuette of a woman who seems to have 'thousands of years of purely sensual, purely unspiritual knowledge behind her'. The higher human impulses: 'the goodness, the holiness, the desire for creation and productive happiness', seem to have disappeared, and this must have led to a sort of death of the human soul suggested by words such as 'corruption', 'dissolution' and 'disintegration'. He goes on to imagine that for the white races this will happen in a different way: destruction through ice and snow and Arctic pitilessness, rather than through the burning heat of the sun. All this obsession with destruction may have been part of Lawrence's reaction to the war. He was writing in 1915–16 when people in England were just beginning to realise the horrifying scale of the slaughter.

But the air now clears a little. Birkin decides that dissolution isn't inevitable for him. There is another way, which is to marry Ursula and have a pure, free union with her. He rushes off to Beldover to ask her to marry him. At the house, the first person he encounters is Ursula's father, so with a rather comic formality he asks him for his daughter's hand. 'I don't know,' says Mr Brangwen, 'she'll please herself – she always has done.' But Ursula refuses to answer, one way or the other. Later on she discusses the proposal with her sister and they agree that Birkin is too much of a preacher and would be impossible to live with. And that settles the matter as far as Gudrun is concerned. But, as so often happens when your friend or your sister agrees with you that you should forget about the man, you start to yearn for him even more. Ursula wants Birkin terribly, but she doesn't want to share him with a philosophical creed. 'She wanted unspeakable intimacies' (wonderful phrase). 'She wanted to have him utterly, finally as her own, oh, so unspeakably, in intimacy. To drink him down – ah, like a life-draught.' Phew, this is heady stuff. And it all began with that cool moonlight on the water.

Wrestling in the library

The next chapter (Chapter 20) is called 'Gladiatorial', and it's the one where Birkin and Gerald improve their man-to-man relationship with a little naked wrestling in Gerald's library. Lawrence's description in words is even more involving than Ken Russell's pictures. He evokes the white flesh, the contrasting bodies, the sudden sounds, the sensations and thoughts of the two men as they struggle until both are exhausted. Gerald, the more powerful of the two, claims to be holding back a little, but he admits that he is impressed by Birkin's different strength. Then the two men have their conversation about the two women. Gerald is pleased to hear that his friend is in love and hopes still to marry Ursula, but says he doubts that he will ever feel real love for a woman himself. Birkin tries to reassure him that there are other ways to fulfilment. 'So long as I feel I've lived, somehow – and I don't care how it is – but I want to feel that –'. Which makes me feel kind of sad for Gerald.

The dying man

Chapter 21 ('Threshold') is of special interest to doctors as it describes the terminal illness of Gerald's father and the differing reactions of his family. His little daughter Winifred is a constant visitor to her daddy's sickroom and it is clear that they are very dear to each other, even as the old man tries to shield her from the knowledge that he is dying. We share some of his thoughts about dying too: he would like to cry out and complain to Gerald, his eldest, and 'shock him out of his composure'. But Gerald is completely repelled by the 'uncleanness' of a death which is out of the person's control. He doesn't want his emotions involved, and yet: 'in some strange way he was a tower of strength to his father'. We might discuss that one at our next terminal care seminar.

Love in Sherwood Forest

We now move on to the chapter in which Ursula takes her courage in both hands and agrees to marry Rupert Birkin, difficult man though he is. Rupert takes her for a drive in the country and shows her three rings with different coloured stones that he has bought for her. Ursula wants to stay out all evening but Birkin says he must be home in time to say goodbye to Hermione. This rouses a terrible jealousy in Ursula's heart. She gets out of the car and has a long rant about Hermione. At first she accuses her of a sham spirituality and 'social passion'. Then, working herself into a fury, she goes on about Hermione being foul and dirty and Birkin enjoying a foul sex life with her. This tirade is amusingly and realistically silenced by the need to say 'Good afternoon' to a passing cyclist. When the quarrel resumes, Ursula throws the rings at him and they fall into the mud. Birkin retrieves them and picks her a flower, a purple-red bell-heather. They kiss and make up. They drive to an inn, have some tea, and in the parlour, by the fire, they embrace in a special way. Ursula kneels in front of Rupert and puts her arms round his loins and her face against his thighs. What is going on here? The sex scenes are by no means as explicit as the ones Lawrence was later to write for Lady Chatterley and Mellors. At first it seems that Ursula is going to give Rupert oral sex, but having read the passage many times I have concluded that this is not the case. The important thing is the stroking of his lumbar region, from which seems to emanate a special kind of god-like male energy, 'stronger than the phallic source'. This experience, both sensual and mystical, has a profound effect on both of them. They decide that they will give up their jobs and run off together. They drive to Sherwood Forest and they make love in the woods, where, Lawrence tells us, they each had their desire fulfilled: 'She was to him what he was to her, the immemorial magnificence of mystic, palpable otherness.' It looks as if their relationship might be going to work out after all.

Death and love

In Chapter 24 ('Death and Love') Gerald's father continues to decline and Gerald finds his feelings very difficult to cope with. For the first time in his life the man of action finds that there is nothing to be done. It seems to be the horror of death itself rather than the loss of his father which is so upsetting for him. Gudrun responds to his distress and comforts him: 'So she relaxed and seemed to melt, to flow into him, as if she were some infinitely warm and precious suffusion filling into his veins, like an intoxicant.' Then his father finally gives up the struggle. The death and the family's reactions are realistically and painfully described. After a few days Gerald finds his loneliness and panic about death unbearable. He stumbles off through the night, heading for Gudrun's house. The front door is unlocked and, taking care not to waken her parents and sister, he creeps up the stairs with mud on his shoes, until he finds Gudrun's bedroom. She welcomes him sleepily and they have sex for the first time. All Gerald's pent-up anguish seems to pour out of him to be contained by Gudrun. He feels relaxed and at peace, and, as Lawrence says, 'like an infant at its mother's breast'. He goes to sleep, the way men do, but Gudrun feels both exhausted and restless. She gazes at the sleeping man with tenderness, but at the same time she feels that there will always be a distance between them.

Marriage or not?

Now it's time for another of Gerald's and Rupert's conversations about women. Birkin is in favour of marriage to one woman for life – but not the conventional domestic cosiness centred on 'home'. There must be something 'additional to marriage' between the man and the woman. Well, we've heard this before, but what does Gerald think? ' "I know," said Gerald, "you believe something like that but I can't feel it, you see." He put his hand on his friend's arm with a sort of deprecating affection. And he smiled as if triumphantly.' And here we share Gerald's silent thoughts. For him, marriage would feel like accepting his place in the social order and thus 'being condemned to live in the mines of the underworld'. He can't conceive of the kind of liberating relationship with a woman that his friend is talking about. Nor can he accept Rupert's offer of an alliance between the two men and subsequently with Gudrun.

The next chapter (Chapter 26, 'The Chair') begins as a pleasant interlude in which Birkin and Ursula, like any engaged couple (don't be fooled), go looking at furniture in the marketplace. They buy an attractive chair but then decide to give it to a conventional working-class couple who are also looking at the stalls. The two couples seem to have a lot in common and Birkin is really nice to them, although they have no idea what sort of person they are talking to. Afterwards, Birkin starts to fret about wanting a close fellowship with Gerald as well as his super-marriage with Ursula. He has really been overcome with a longing for Gerald, whom he seems to be losing. 'Do I want,' he asks Ursula, 'a relationship in the ultimate of him and me – or don't I?' Well, what would you say? 'She looked at him for a long time with her strange bright eyes but she did not answer.'

Back home, Ursula tells Gudrun and her parents that she is going to be married to Birkin the following day. Her father is very angry and ends up hitting her. Ursula runs off to join Birkin and stays the night with him. They are married the next day in a civil ceremony. Later, Birkin proposes that all four of them should go away together. Gerald agrees, but Gudrun has not yet been consulted. Later, Ursula goes back to get her possessions from the cold, empty family house from which their parents have now moved. They discuss whether they would want the sort of life their parents have had – bringing up children in a home – and decide definitely not. Gudrun broods about herself and Gerald. She loves him but when she compares her love with Ursula's 'her soul was jealous, unsatisfied'. And she is cross when Ursula tells her that Gerald has agreed to Birkin's proposal for a joint holiday. She feels she is being treated no differently from one of Gerald's casual London pick-ups. In the brief chapter that follows, before they get on the boat train, she and Gerald pay a last visit to the Chelsea artists' sleazy café ('The Pompadour'). Gudrun over-hears one of their artist friends reading mockingly from one of Birkin's letters to the great amusement of the company. Gudrun is furious: she snatches the letter and walks out with it before anyone can stop her. It's a brave gesture showing Gudrun's better side; we feel that she has rescued Birkin from the clutches of the London gang, who don't appreciate him, and enabled him to escape with Ursula.

Four go on holiday together

The four travellers cross the channel and then go by train from Brussels to Basle and then by a small mountain railway to the high-est accessible part of the Austrian Alps. There is snow everywhere and Lawrence describes it beautifully. But Gudrun is rather shocked, perhaps because blonde Nordic Gerald has brought her into his icy heartland. '"My God, Jerry," she said, turning to Gerald with sudden intimacy, "you've done it now."' That is the only time she calls him Jerry. By the time they reach the little hotel where they are going to stay, Gudrun is enjoying the experience. Gerald kisses her passionately and says he will always love her – but Gudrun, looking at him is 'silent and remote'. She feels herself falling away from him. She looks at Ursula and Rupert sitting together and again she feels jealous of them.

They go into the hotel and are introduced to the other guests, a party of Germans, including artists, students and a professor with his two teenage daughters. They have dinner; there is singing and dancing. Ursula dances with Birkin and under the feel of his hands has a strange experience in which she finds him, at first, quite frightening. She feels that they are going to do 'degrading' and 'bestial' things together in bed. But then she thinks: who cares? 'How good it was to be really shameful! There would be no shameful thing she had not experienced.' What shameful things? The details are left to our imagination, but intercourse from behind is almost certainly involved. All right, buggery. You made me say it. Lawrence regarded this popular sexual variation as 'degrading'. However, when it was practised by the right people, it could help to bring about dissolution, leading to rebirth and a new world order. It's difficult to see exactly how this will come to pass but it's a recurring theme in Birkin's (and Lawrence's) philosophy.

Meanwhile Gudrun, who has been watching Gerald dancing with the professor's daughter, has a sudden revelation that he is 'naturally promiscuous'. She decides that there is going to be a battle between them and that she is going to win. Later on, she imagines herself as the quietly powerful wife of a successful man. She will be at his side while he restructures British industry, or becomes a great politician like Bismarck (remember Bismarck the rabbit?). He is the perfect instrument. But for what? She is quickly disillusioned with this vision of Gerald. She looks at him fondly and decides that his true value is to provide her with a few 'perfect moments'. 'You've convinced me,' she says as he wakes up. And he kisses her, but he doesn't understand.

Parting of the ways

Then comes a crucial section where we are introduced to one of the German artists in the hotel, a man called Loerke. He is 'a small dark skinned man with full eyes, an odd creature, like a child, and like a troll, quick, detached'. Gudrun is interested in him because he is a sculptor. And she is intrigued by his appearance, like a little old man or a gnome. Ursula is attracted to him too. He tells all four of them about a frieze he is sculpting to adorn a factory. The men both dislike him instinctively. But Birkin has a strange, grudging admiration for him as well. He sees him as corrupt and degraded. As we know, he believes that human society must somehow come to an end through moral decline and catastrophe before the new world order can emerge. So filth and degradation are good. He tells Gerald that Loerke 'lives like a rat in the sewers of corruption, just where it falls over into the bottomless pit. He's farther on than we are. He hates the ideal more acutely. … I expect he is a Jew – or part Jewish.' Oh dear, there is Lawrence's anti-Semitism, coming out embarrassingly. I try to remind myself that one of his best friends was the Jewish artist Mark Gertler. What do you say if your friend comes out with that kind of rubbish? I hope that Gertler just hit him. To make sure that we really despise and loathe poor old Loerke, we are told that he uses adolescent girls as models and is practically a paedophile (or at least a teenophile). We shall see Loerke's pivotal role in the conclusion of the story in the next chapter. But now it is time for our couples to part. Ursula wants to get away from the ice and snow and head for the warm south. Birkin agrees that they will leave. She and Gudrun have a parting talk and Gudrun makes her a present of some of her best coloured stockings. ('One gets the greatest joy of all out of really lovely stockings,' says Ursula.)

Gudrun asks her sister if she feels that she is 'going-away-for-ever, never-to-return, sort of thing?' 'I only know we are going somewhere,' says Ursula. And she is *very* glad'. Has she begun to share Birkin's belief that there is something even better beyond love? Well, partly. Gudrun doesn't understand but she wishes her sister well. Birkin says goodbye to Gerald and his last words are: 'I've loved you as well as Gudrun, don't forget.' But Gerald still doesn't get it. I love Gerald too. He is so wonderfully bemused when confronted with the higher Lawrentian ideals.

Death in the Alps

And so Gudrun and Gerald are left alone in the alpine hotel. Gudrun forces Gerald to admit that he doesn't love her, has never loved her. He says he doesn't know what love means. Then she wants him to say 'I love you', even if he doesn't mean it – and he obliges. They make love again: they still have plenty of desire for each other – but afterwards each thinks about getting free of the other. Gerald's thoughts are very troubled. He wants to be self-sufficient, closed up and protected. But Gudrun has opened him up and 'a strange rent had been torn in him'. The wound is both painful and joyful and he doesn't altogether want it to heal. Gudrun also feels torn open. And Gerald is now so tortured that he is thinking about killing her. Things are not going well here. And to make matters worse, Loerke, the creepy sculptor, continues to take an interest in Gudrun. He is greatly encouraged when she tells him she is not married to Gerald. Gudrun enjoys talking art with Loerke in a way that she could never do with Gerald. Life with him would be as mechanical and repetitive as the industrial machinery that he commands. At the same time, he is like a great baby who needs to be lulled to sleep. Meanwhile Gerald keeps having worrying impulses to strangle Gudrun. In the morning, she tells him that she will be leaving the next day. She and Loerke go out into the snow and have a picnic. Then things get scary. 'Suddenly, they were aware of a vague white figure near them.' It is Gerald. He knocks Loerke down and seizes Gudrun round the throat. It seems as if he will really strangle her. Then suddenly he relaxes his grip and stumbles away, up the snow slope towards the summit. We get the feeling now that he just wants to die. He loses himself, loses consciousness and dies in the snow.

The last chapter

Gerald's body is discovered and brought back to the hotel. Ursula and Birkin return. Birkin goes to look at the body of his friend. He is horrified by the icy coldness of the dead man. He goes out to the snow slope to see where the death occurred and finds that there is a fixed rope along which Gerald might have dragged himself to safety. We wonder if he missed his chance to use Birkin's offer of brotherhood as a lifeline. Birkin's grief for Gerald is very moving. Ursula stands watching him jealously and says, 'You've got me.' And later: 'Aren't I enough for you?' And so they are at odds once again. Happy as he is with Ursula, Birkin also wanted 'eternal union with a man too: another kind of love'. They disagree. But they survive, and we get the impression that they will stay with each other, just as Lawrence and his wife, Frieda, stayed together. Perhaps a different part of Lawrence died with Gerald in the ice and snow. The music I hear now is Siegfried's funeral march from Wagner's *Götterdammerung*.

Retrospective

I am standing in the snow at the end of *Women in Love*, still stunned by the tragedy of Gerald's death. I am wondering what will happen to Gudrun. I am partly solaced by the thought that Ursula and Rupert might stay together, and learn to understand and tolerate each other. As I walk slowly back to my hotel through the crisp snow, I reflect on the experience of reading and living with *Women in Love* as follows.

It's a beautiful book. Nobody else can write like Lawrence at his best. The poetic descriptions (the moon, the lake at night with the boats and the lanterns, the animals, the snow and ice at the climax) are all wonderful. There are also very subtle descriptions of the lovers' states of mind as they veer between love and hate, desire and detachment, affection and contempt. What about Birkin's ideas, Lawrence's ideas? How seriously are we to take them? Do they make sense or are they simply strange and stirring? Are they dangerous? They are certainly an essential part of the plot, but Birkin is very much more than a mouthpiece for Lawrence's gospel. And he comes in for a good deal of mockery, not just from Ursula but from the author himself. I found it helpful to try to understand what he is getting at and perhaps see his ideas in the context of the time in which Lawrence was living. But, in the end, the characters, the story and the lyrical poetry of the writing are more important.

A doctor writes

I want to take a last look at the book as a doctor. My diagnosis of Gerald is that he is suffering from depression. Do you agree?

Maybe some Prozac would have helped. But he also needed someone who could have warmed his chilly, frozen soul back into life. Gudrun can't do it, because she is also short of inner warmth. She responds joyfully to Gerald's sexual aggression, but she can't begin to accept and contain his grief. The most she can do is to tear a gash that exposes his feelings and his neediness. But that isn't the way; it's too brutal. He really needs a patient and concerned therapist to stay with him and help him not to be afraid of feeling dependent. I am less clear about Birkin's psychopathology. Maybe he is just a man possessed by the excitement of a developing vision about how one should live and love in the world. Not mad, but difficult to live with. I think he should definitely try to be a writer: it will channel his energies more productively. And I think Ursula will manage to be a therapeutic wife for Rupert, much as Frieda was in real life for Lawrence. She will listen to him, make fun of him and fight with him, but she will love and respect him and stay with him all his life as wife and mother. Did Lawrence have a therapist? He was certainly interested in psychoanalysis and was friendly with some eminent English analysts. He even wrote about psychoanalysis and the unconscious mind, though he soon veered off into his own preoccupations. No, I think he just had Frieda. And what about Rupert's need for Gerald? Maybe that is something about needing a father as well as a mother. Or if that is too psychoanalytic, about a man's need to have a warm and close relationship with a different kind of man, regardless of their sexual orientation.

Finally ...

I have spent a long time with this book. Its music appealed to me instantly but it took me longer to get to know the characters and to appreciate their feelings. Still, it was well worth the effort, and Rupert, Gerald, Ursula and Gudrun have become permanent residents of my inner world of literature. I hope that you too will read and enjoy *Women in Love*, and that, if you are not already Lawrentians, it will open some windows for you onto a new literary landscape.

The text

Women in Love is available in the Penguin Modern Classics series, edited by David Farmer, Lindeth Vasey and John Worthen, with an introduction and notes by Mark Kinkead-Weekes.

13

A Passage to India

by EM Forster (1924)

Edward Morgan Forster (always known as EM) was born in 1879 and wrote most of his novels between 1905 and 1910. These include *Howards End* and *A Room with a View,* both of which have been turned into successful British films in the past few years. *A Passage to India* has also been filmed, but many years earlier. I first read it when I was a student; I remember being gripped by the conflict between the supercilious English colonial administrators and the defiant Indians who had to suffer under the brutal insensitivity of their rulers. I felt indignant at the way young Dr Aziz (yes, this is another novel with a doctor hero) was treated and I longed for him to be vindicated and India to be free.

Now that I've read it again, 40 years later, it seems a very different book, much more complicated and rather mysterious. I wondered how much India and the relations between the different branches of the human race had changed. I wondered if my own attitudes had changed. And I wondered, as I usually do, what sort of person had written the book.

So, before we start, let me tell you what I know about Forster – which is not very much. His father died within a year of his birth and he was brought up by his mother. After an unhappy time at a public school he went to Cambridge University, where he made friends with lots of other people who liked books and ideas. At some stage during his school or college years he must have realised that he was gay. In 1913 he wrote a homosexual novel (*Maurice*) and circulated it privately. It was not finally published until after his death, when his sexual inclinations could become public knowledge. He didn't marry or have children. I don't know if he ever had a long-term partner. He seems to have fallen in love with a young Indian man called Syed Ross Masood, whom he tutored after he left Cambridge. Syed (to whom *A Passage to India* is dedicated) was straight, so there was no romance, but they remained friends for many years.

Forster started *A Passage to India* after his first visit to India in 1912, but he seems to have got stuck and abandoned it until after the end of the First World War. He finally completed it in 1922–24, and it is generally regarded as his finest achievement. Strangely, he then ran out of creative inspiration and wrote no more novels, although he survived until 1971. He was an academic and literary critic for most of these years and he wrote some travel books and essays. My impression after reading some of his essays (*Two Cheers for Democracy*, 1951) is that he must have been a nice man, a very decent man. He loved music and literature and he hated prejudice and injustice. He believed that personal relationships were more important than politics and ideology. 'Tolerance, good temper and sympathy – they are what matter really,' he said. He was also the man who wrote 'Only connect ...' as the epigraph to *Howard's End*.

First impressions

The book begins with a bird's-eye view of the fictitious Indian city of Chandrapore. As if in a helicopter, we swoop from the river Ganges over the dull, mean streets of the poorer (Indian) quarter and the more substantial houses of the Eurasian quarter. We observe the Maidan (polo lawn for British officers) and the hospital. Then, on higher ground, comes the 'Civil Station' where the English folk live in their neatly arranged bungalows. From here, we are told, the squalid houses down below are hidden by the trees and the whole town looks like a garden. Everywhere the land is flat – except in the south, where the Marabar Hills appear like 'a group of fists and fingers thrust up through the soil'. These hills contain some strange caves in which an unpleasant incident will violently alter the lives of all the main characters – but that comes later. After a troubled gaze at those pregnant hills, Chapter 1 ends suddenly and we are deposited down in the lower town just in time to meet Dr Aziz and his friends.

Aziz and his friends

Aziz seems to be about 30. He is a doctor who works at the local hospital, and his two chums are both barristers. They are all educated men and the elder barrister (Hamidullah) was at Cambridge. As they wait for the servants to prepare their dinner they pass round the hookah and have a discussion about whether it is possible to be friends with an Englishman. Hamidullah thinks it is possible, but only in England. When they first arrive in India the English 'behave like gentlemen', but soon the older residents tell them 'it won't do' to be friendly to the Indians. After two years, says Hamidullah, they are all the same. And the women are even worse: they only take six months to adopt the insulting, superior, colonial attitude. After dinner, the three men visit Hamidullah's wife, who is in 'purdah' and doesn't come out in public. We realise, if we haven't already noticed from their names, that they are all Muslims. From the conversation with Mrs Hamidullah we learn that Aziz is a widower who has three young children in the care of his late wife's mother. Later in the evening, a messenger summons Dr Aziz to the house of his boss, the English Major Callendar. Aziz wonders whether there is a case he wants to discuss or whether Callendar is deliberately interrupting their dinner hour 'just to show his power'. Their discussion is overshadowed by their resentment at the arrogant and contemptuous way in which their English masters treat them; the fact that the Indians are professional colleagues seems to make no difference. Poor Aziz pedals off obediently on his bike, has a puncture and hires a 'tonga' (a sort of rickshaw). When he arrives, Major Callendar is out and his tonga is promptly commandeered by Mrs Callendar and her friend: two typically toffee-nosed English ladies. Aziz is terribly polite and courteous to them but they ignore him. He is an Indian, but not one of their household servants, and therefore invisible. Despite all these insults Aziz has a paradoxical admiration for English people and is just desperate to win their approval. It's pathetic and a bit embarrassing for us readers. Why does he do it? Is that how educated Indians behaved in 1912? Do they still feel the same way? These questions about race and relationships will recur constantly throughout the book.

Meeting in a mosque

On his way home, Aziz sits down for a rest in the courtyard of a mosque. He is suddenly aware of the presence of an elderly Englishwoman with a red face and white hair. This is Mrs Moore, who has recently arrived from England to visit her son Ronny, who is the City Magistrate in Chandrapore. At first Aziz scolds Mrs Moore for coming into a holy place with her shoes on. Then he discovers that she has taken them off and he apologises. They fall into a friendly, open conversation and he makes the happy discovery that she is totally free of racist prejudices. Encouraged by her hints that she is not too keen on Mrs Callendar either, he lets himself go in a little outburst of pain about the way he has been treated, is always treated by the Brits. She invites him to come and see her at 'the Club': he has to tell her that Indians are not allowed in the Club – not even as guests.

Members only

In Chapter 3, Forster takes English readers back into the safety of their own territory – to see how they like it. We are in the Club at Chandrapore and everyone has a white skin – except the servants. The first person we meet is Adela Quested, a young girl who has just arrived from England with Mrs Moore. The idea is that she should marry Mrs Moore's son, Ronny, whom she already knows slightly. Adela says 'I want to see the real India' – by which she means she would like to meet some Indian people. Mrs Moore agrees with her, but the other women are amused and slightly repelled by the idea of mixing socially with the natives. 'They don't respect you any more,' says one colonial wife and another says: 'They give me the creeps.' Mr Turton, the collector (chief administrator), offers to hold a party to which some suitable Indians will be invited for Mrs Moore's benefit. (Perhaps she will see sense when she knows what they are like.) On the way home, Mrs Moore tells Ronny and Adela about her meeting with a nice young Muslim doctor at the mosque. Adela is thrilled but Ronny is very disapproving. His view of the encounter is that Aziz was being impertinent, especially in expressing his disapproval of his boss, Major Callendar. 'It's the educated native's latest dodge. They used to cringe but the younger generation believe in a show of manly independence.' His mother tells him that he never used to judge people like that at home and Ronny replies rather abruptly: 'India isn't home'. He begins to worry that his mother will influence Adela who, if she is going to be his wife, has to have all the right prejudices to fit in with the other colonial wives.

By this stage, we feel that the battle lines are drawn up and we know which side we are on. We are with Mrs Moore, Adela and the Indians, and against the cold-blooded, racist British imperialists. We needn't feel disloyal because we British are not like that any more. Or are we? How do we treat our own citizens of Asian or African origin? Is racism no longer a problem? These questions will continue to pop up and disturb us. Meanwhile, as Mrs Moore is about to hang up her cloak for the night, she observes a little wasp with long yellow legs, asleep on the tip of the clothes peg. The night outside is full of jungle noises but the wasp sleeps peacefully. '"Pretty dear," said Mrs Moore to the wasp. He did not wake but her voice floated out to swell the night's uneasiness.' Now I couldn't tell you why Mr Forster ends this chapter with Mrs Moore's salute to the Indian wasp: but it's an image which lingers in my memory and seems to be very important.

The party to meet the Indians duly takes place and it's not a great success. It is called a 'Bridge Party', not because anyone plays cards, but because it is supposed to bridge the gulf between East and West. But the English hosts and particularly the women prefer to stay on their side of the bridge and not get too close. The exception is Mr Fielding, who is head teacher of the Government College, where his pupils are young Indians. Fielding is a bachelor in his forties and he is refreshingly free of racism. Perhaps he represents Forster himself. He invites Mrs Moore and Adela to come to tea at his house and meet some Indians properly – including Dr Aziz.

Getting to know Dr Aziz

In the next chapter we learn a bit more about Aziz and his past history. He has stayed away from the party, partly because he can't stand most of the English and partly because it's the anniversary of his wife's death. He had objected to the arranged marriage initially, but began to love his wife after their first child was born. She died giving birth to their third child and now he keeps a picture of her in his drawer. When he looks at the picture he cries, but he finds it difficult to remember her. He wonders if they will meet again after death. Faith tells him they will, but like everyone's his faith wavers. He feels lost and depressed about his personal and professional future. After tea, he cheers up a bit, borrows a pony and rides off to the Maidan, where he finds a British subaltern practising polo. He invites Aziz to join in and they play together happily for a short time, racial differences forgotten. 'If only they were all like that,' thinks Aziz. Later we discover that this subaltern is as bad as all the rest. In this chapter we get to know Aziz much better: he is an individual and he is complicated; by no means a mere symbol of the oppressed Indian. He is looking forward to tea with Fielding, whom he has not so far met.

A multicultural tea party

When Aziz arrives, Fielding is still in the bathroom and he shouts out 'Please make yourself at home.' Aziz does so and their relationship develops very happily from this natural, spontaneous beginning. With this Englishman, Aziz is able to relax; he is at his best: witty, charming, considerate and full of fun, as he chats away happily. He lends Fielding a collar stud and helps him to put it in. When Mrs Moore and Adela arrive things continue to go well, and Aziz tries to explain Indian customs to the two women. He tells them his idea of justice, which is to give the criminal another chance because gaol will only make him worse. Forster notes that Aziz is tender to everyone (except a few enemies). He is even tender to the English because 'they could not help being so cold and odd and circulating like an ice-stream through his land'. The tea party is punctuated by the arrival of an eminent and eccentric Hindu Brahmin, Professor Godbole, who is also a teacher at Fielding's college. The elderly professor sits apart from the others, eats his special food and smiles enigmatically. He seems to represent the mystical side of India, which the pragmatic, earth-bound English will never understand. Aziz invites everyone on an expedition to see the famous Marabar caves. He asks the professor to describe the wonders of the caves, but the old man disappoints him by saying they are quite ordinary. Then young Ronny arrives and tries to drag the women away. He makes no attempt to hide his disapproval of their choice of company. Just before they leave, Professor Godbole announces that he is going to sing: and we get a vivid glimpse of the strangeness and wonder of spiritual India. After the song he tries to tell the women what it was about. The God Krishna appears to a group of milkmaids and one of them asks him to come – but he refuses to come. '"I say to Him, Come, come, come, come, come, come. He neglects to come."' The idea of the old professor role-playing an amorous milkmaiden is very funny; at the same time, we are aware of our own Gods, persistently neglecting to come.

On the way home, Adela tells Ronny that she is not going to marry him after all (and we readers secretly celebrate). But then they are involved in a minor road accident, they hold hands in the back of the car and soon the engagement is on again. This is an entertaining episode, which I must leave you to read for yourselves, because we must now move on to Part Two of the book and the expedition to the Marabar caves.

Don't go into those caves

Part Two opens with a lyrical geology of Southern India, leading to a description of the caves. There are lots and lots of them, all very much the same. Each has an entrance tunnel eight feet long, leading to a dark circular chamber twenty feet in diameter. If you strike a match in a cave you get a reflected image of the flame because the spherical walls are highly polished. There are said to be hundreds of sealed chambers without entrance tunnels. One of these is rumoured to be inside a huge boulder which balances and sways on the summit of the Kawa Dol, the highest of the Marabar peaks. So our friends are about to visit some very spooky caves.

The expedition starts rather badly when Fielding and Professor Godbole are delayed by the professor's prayers and miss the train. Still, the ladies enjoy the scenic journey and Adela makes plans for her forthcoming life in India as Ronny's wife. At the end of the line, Aziz has ordered an elephant to take them the rest of the way up to the caves. As the elephant plods higher, everything becomes quiet and the light plays tricks: is that a black snake or just a tree branch? They stop for breakfast (tea and poached eggs) and Aziz chats happily with his English lady friends about the Mogul emperors. Then they go into the first cave and Mrs Moore has a really terrifying experience. In fact, she will never be the same again, for reasons which are difficult to grasp. The cave is full of people, it's dark and it smells bad. She can't breathe and people are crushing her. Some nasty fleshy thing settles on her mouth. Ugh! Actually it turns out to be only a baby, astride its mother's hip. The whole thing is like a panic attack. But the worst part is the echo she hears in the cave. It goes 'ou-boum' (according to Forster), and it tells poor Mrs Moore that nothing in human existence is really worthwhile, nothing you can do will make any difference and there is only despair. She sits down on the ground and no longer wants to write to her children or communicate with anyone. This is very strange and dismaying for the reader. Is she overwhelmed by the vast, unfeeling universe? Is she clinically depressed all of a sudden? Whatever it is, Mrs Moore's kindness, tolerance and sympathy have all ceased to function. Only her honesty remains.

Now we leave Mrs Moore sitting on the ground and join Aziz and Adela on their way to the second cave. Adela is still thinking about marriage – and love. She and Ronny do not love each other, she tells herself. Then she asks Aziz if he is married. Aziz says,

'"Yes, indeed, do come and see my wife" – for he felt it more artistic to have his wife alive for a moment.' They talk about his children and then Adela asks if he has more than one wife (because Mrs Turton, the collector's wife, says that Mohammedans always insist on their full four). Poor Aziz is totally taken aback and deeply offended. He plunges into the nearest cave to recover his cool; Adela wanders into another cave, still thinking about marriage (or perhaps about sex).

When she comes out, all hell is let loose. She, too, has had a seriously bad experience in one of those womb-like caves. She flees in terror down the hill and is taken home by a young Englishwoman who has just arrived on the scene by car, together with Fielding. Aziz finds her field glasses lying outside a cave with the strap broken – and puts them in his pocket. When the others arrive home on the train, they are met by Mr Haq, the Indian police inspector, who says he has orders to put Aziz under arrest!

The charge

What is he supposed to have done? The charge is 'That he followed the girl into the cave and made insulting advances'. She says that she hit at him with her field glasses, he grabbed them and when the strap broke she was able to escape. And, sure enough, when they search him, there are the field glasses in his pocket, with the strap broken. Fielding, who doesn't believe a word of it, tries to intercede with the collector, who has also come to the station to watch the arrest. There must have been a mistake, Fielding protests. But the collector observes bitterly that the mistake is for English people and Indians to 'attempt to be intimate socially'. According to him and his 25 years' experience, it always leads to disaster. But Aziz is refused bail and is led off weeping. Fielding is refused permission to see him. The English colony all close ranks to defend the honour of their injured female member. Fielding finds himself alienated from his fellow countrymen and siding with Aziz's Indian friends in their campaign to free him and to clear his name. There are some exciting scenes at the Club when Fielding stoutly maintains that Aziz is innocent and refuses to stand up with the others when Ronny (who is felt to have been equally injured) comes into the room. Down in the city there are angry rumblings as the news spreads of an outrageous wrongful arrest: there are fears at the Club of rioting and insurrection by the natives. Just what they were here to prevent.

But what really happened in Adela's cave? Her own account to Ronny is that she scratched the wall of the cave to start an echo. Then a shadow fell across the entrance of the cave, she hit at someone she took to be Aziz with her glasses, he pulled her by the strap, the strap broke and she escaped. She tumbled down the hill and was impaled by lots of cactus thorns. And the sound of the echo had remained in her head ever since. You will remember that she was thinking about marriage when she went into the cave, so perhaps the strange atmosphere and the weird echo induced a sexual hallucination which she took for reality.

What has happened to Mrs Moore?

What about Mrs Moore, Ronny's mother? Adela looks to her for sympathy and support while Ronny is expecting her to give evidence for the prosecution at the forthcoming trial. Both are disappointed, for, as we have seen, Mrs Moore is now totally switched off. 'She seemed to say: "Am I to be bothered for ever?" Her Christian tenderness had gone, or had developed into a hardness, a just irritation against the human race.' Even though she believes that Aziz is innocent she seems to feel totally detached from the whole business and refuses to give evidence at the trial either for him or against him. She seems to be preoccupied with a feeling that she has become a bad person herself. 'I used to be good with the children growing up, also I meet this young man in his mosque, I wanted him to be happy. Good, happy, small people. They do not exist, they were a dream .... But I will not help you torture him for what he never did.'

It's hard to know what to make of this change in Mrs Moore. Have the evil spirits in the cave got into her brain? Is it some sort of dementia with depression that is afflicting her? Whatever it is, the effect is quite shattering and totally believable.

The trial

And so Dr Aziz is put on trial for assaulting or insulting a young white woman. Although Ronny is City Magistrate, everyone accepts that he cannot try the case himself. Mr Das, his Indian deputy, is in the chair and desperately anxious to keep the proceedings under control. We see the crowded courtroom mainly from Adela's point of view, and the first person she notices is the magnificent muscular figure of the punkah-wallah, the Indian man whose job it is to operate a huge fan which cools everyone except himself. You will notice that, at the end of the courtroom drama, the last person we see is also the punkah-wallah, who has been present throughout, and been totally unperturbed by the proceedings, like the vast country of India itself.

Naturally, the English community find it very difficult to submit to the authority of an Indian magistrate. They all want to sit on the platform and get very cross when, in response to an appeal from Mr Amritrao, the eminent barrister Aziz's friends have brought in to defend him, they are told to go back down again. Even so, they keep shouting out and interrupting the proceedings as though they were really in charge and not Mr Das. The defence expect Mrs Moore to be available to give evidence and are outraged when they learn that she has already left for England. The junior Counsel, Aziz's friend Mahmoud Ali, gets so upset that he rushes out of the court. Fortunately, the more detached Mr Amritrao remains at his post.

I am not going to disclose the outcome of the trial because that would deprive you of the suspense of reading it for yourselves. When it is over, the relationship between Aziz and Fielding continues to develop but it is not without painful misunderstandings. Soon afterwards, Cyril (yes, that is Fielding's first name) returns to England, where Aziz is convinced he will marry Adela.

Part Three: Temple

Let us now have a brief look at the surprising third part of the novel before we finish this account. Two years have passed and the scene has moved to the independent Indian state of Mau, where Professor Godbole has taken up the post of Minister of Education at the court of the Rajah. Aziz and his troubles seem to be miles away and we are in the middle of an important Hindu religious ceremony, with the professor presiding. The ceremony takes place in the ruler's palace and it is beautifully described. Forster wants us to know that, compared with a Western religious occasion, everything seems muddled and confused and lacking in focus. It is also colourful, noisy, wonderful, uplifting and awe-inspiring. They are celebrating the birth of Shri Krishna, who is the embodiment of Infinite Love and will save the world. At the end of the chapter, Godbole suddenly remembers Mrs Moore and wishes he could make the God come to her. But he is aware that his capacities are very small. '"One old Englishwoman and one little, little wasp,"' he thinks to himself. There's that wasp again!

All this is very beautiful and mysterious but incapable of logical explanation. In the last few chapters, there are more Hindu ceremonies and a final meeting between Aziz and Cyril Fielding (who *is* married, but not to Adela Quested). They go for a horse ride together through the jungles of Mau. They discuss all the things that friends talk about: the past, the future, their differing political views, their own relationship. Their conversation is honest, warm, humorous, sometimes belligerent. Aziz says he wants the English to clear out of India. He has a vision of an India in which all Hindus, Muslims and Sikhs will be united. Fielding derides this as a possibility and Aziz says, '"We may hate one another but we hate you most ... if it's fifty or five hundred years we shall get rid of you ... yes, we shall drive every blasted Englishman into the sea and then" – he rode against him furiously – "and then," he concluded, half kissing him, "you and I shall be friends."' Fielding asks why they can't be friends now. But the horses swerve and pull them apart.

I find this an exciting and moving ending. It also reflects Forster's belief that personal loyalties are more important than political ones. I close the book thinking about his love for India, his love for a young Indian friend and his life which, although satisfying in many ways, probably lacked the fulfilment of a deep and lasting intimate relationship.

The text

A Passage to India by EM Forster was first published in 1924 and is available in the Penguin edition, with an introduction by Oliver Stallybrass.

Postscript: East is East and West is West: will the twain ever meet? by Professor Aziz Sheikh

A Passage to India, widely acknowledged to be EM Forster's finest contribution to English literature, is a thoughtful and sensitive exploration into the highly complex subject of human relationships. He considers the subject from a number of perspectives and dimensions – and herein lies the great strength of his work – ranging from relationships with the metaphysical world (it is no coincidence that two of the three parts reflect sacred institutions), with the awe-inspiring and at times incomprehensible inanimate world (the Marabar caves, for example), and between distinct human cultures and civilisations (British and Indian; secular and theistic). And though these complex inter-relationships are all undoubtedly important, betraying his own struggle to make sense of the world around him, there is no mistaking the fact that, of even greater importance to the author, is the question of *individual* relationships.

How much needs to be overcome and endured if *true* friendship between two human beings is to flourish? This is the question that reverberates throughout this beautifully crafted work, a question that is explored through the characters of Cyril Fielding and Dr Aziz, thought by many commentators to personify, to some extent at least, Forster himself and his close friend Syed Ross Masood, whom he met while in India. It is, then, perhaps unsurprising to many contemporary readers that it is to Masood that Forster dedicated this book. In order to make fuller sense of the significance of this gesture, however, and indeed the central themes and characters in this book, there is a need, I believe, to appreciate the wider political and social climate within which this work was written. Such considerations are essential if we are to make any attempt to consider how Forster might view relationships between the rich variety of races and religious groups that have now – whether through choice or circumstance – made their home in his country of birth.

Britain's passage to India: birth of an empire

The Anglo-Indian relationship dates back at least to the beginning of the seventeenth century when the British-based East India Company began trading with India. Relationships were at first amicable, with British sailors actively encouraged to assimilate and integrate with Indian society. A sharp downturn in trust, however, occurred in 1750, following rumours that a group of British travellers had been suffocated by their hosts in an event that was subsequently to become known as 'The Black Hole of Calcutta'. In order to avenge this incident, a group of British soldiers set sail for India, under the stewardship of Robert Clive, on an expedition that was to culminate in the seizure of Bengal. And so began a chain of events that led, over the next century or so, to the East India Company successfully procuring large stretches of Indian territory and in so doing, subjugating the natives. What motivated this hardening of attitudes towards the Indians? Surely, an isolated incident, no matter how horrific, could not in itself have been sufficient to sustain a systematic colonial movement?

To make sense of the changing mentality of the British, one needs to take a broader historical perspective and look at social developments in Britain. There was, at around the same time, a newly found confidence within European society, inspired, not so much by claims to a divine right to rule (although this too was important), but by rapid and sustained material and technological progress – a period that was later known as the Industrial Revolution. These material advances were, or so it seemed to many, just desert for a morally upright civilisation. And it was widely perceived as a moral obligation on such a society to share its success with the less privileged. The imperial apologist Kipling would later justify American conduct in the Philippines by referring to the duty to discharge 'the white man's burden'; other writers took up the phrase to celebrate the ignoble imperialist period of British history.

The Jewel in the Crown

The 'mutiny' of 1857, in which the Indians tried unsuccessfully to rid themselves of the parasite that had now infested much of their land, was the catalyst formally to transfer control of India from the East India Company to the British Crown. With the additional sense of superiority provided by social Darwinism, European nations, and Britain in particular, pursued a 'legitimate and just' expansion drive. Such sentiments are clearly evident in the writings from this time; consider for example Brigadier General John Jacob's now infamous communication to his troops:

> We hold India, then, by being in reality, as in reputation, a superior race to the Asiatic; and if this moral superiority did not exist, we should not, and could not, retain the country for one week. If then, we are really a morally superior race, governed by higher motives and possessing higher attributes than the Asiatics, the more the natives of India are able to understand us, and the more we improve their capacity for so understanding, the firmer will become our power. Away, then with the assumption of equality, and let us accept our true position of a dominant race.

After successfully conquering the lands of the impoverished, the British Government, chastened by the 'mutiny' of those they were attempting to civilise, considered new strategies with which to maintain their hegemony. And so was formulated the policy of 'divide and rule', driving once cordial neighbouring communities into intractable cycles of recrimination and violence by successfully sowing the seeds of suspicion, distrust and envy. The policy reaped dividends, playing a key role in the maintenance of an empire that, at its height, spanned four continents. Of all Britain's military successes, India, however, remained the most prized, and it is not insignificant that in 1876, at Disraeli's instigation, the title of Empress of India was conferred on Queen Victoria.

Anglo-Indian relationships: might is right and right is might

Why, despite his suffering an almost daily barrage of insult, did Dr Aziz in EM Forster's book, persist in his hopeless attempts to win the approval of the British? Were his actions typical of those of educated Indians at the time? Have things changed or does the same mentality still exist? These are uncomfortable questions that confront many contemporary Western readers of *A Passage to India*.

Making sense of Dr Aziz is not easy, but the preceding discussion will, I hope, have conveyed something of the oppressive climate into which he was born. His own Muslim culture, once dominant and proud, was also on a sharp decline, adding greatly to his sense of inferiority and impotence. Confronted by such circumstances, and with no clear way out of the abyss in which he found himself, most would, I suspect, have followed suit and capitulated to leading a life that amounted to little more than obedience to their masters' whims. Fear is, and remains, a most potent driving force. Witness, for example, how successive British and European governments insist on riding in tandem with the new dominant culture – whether right or wrong – as it ruthlessly pursues its ambition to create its own New World Order. 'Might is right' remains for most individuals and cultures a proverbial truth, and Dr Aziz's behaviour, alas, proved true to this rule.

The making of the 'Brown Sahib'

But why the 'paradoxical admiration for English people'? Once again, there is a need to turn to the history of the Indian subcontinent and Anglo-Indian relationships if we are to make any sense of Aziz's, at times, seemingly bizarre behaviour. It was Thomas Babington Macaulay, one of the high priests of Victorian European humanism, who set in motion a stratagem from which much of the ex-colonised world has still to recover. In order to realise her interests, Britain would, he noted in his Minute of Education in 1853, create an Indian junior elite: 'A class of persons, Indian in blood and colour but English in taste, in opinions, in morals and in intellect.' This stratagem was vigorously pursued through systematically destroying and dismantling religious institutions, native languages, traditional educational models and family values or, in other words, the very edifices of indigenous tradition and culture.

Dr Aziz, like many of his Western-educated contemporaries, suffered from 'Macaulay syndrome'; those of South Asian origin often describe those afflicted with this malady as 'coconuts' – brown on the outside but white on the inside. Dr Aziz betrays his ailment on innumerable occasions during the course of his own passage to recovery; most telling, perhaps, is when the culturally naive Adela Quested, during the infamous expedition to the Marabar caves, enquires of her guide 'Have you one wife or more than one?' The sense of revulsion felt by Dr Aziz at being posed such a question is both acute and intense. For here is a man who sees little wrong in arranging visits to a brothel in Calcutta – an anathema to the traditional Muslim mind – yet finds loathsome the very idea of responsible and lifelong union through polygamous matrimony. Forster brilliantly conveys Dr Aziz's almost complete detachment from his own Muslim roots by noting: 'If she had said, "Do you worship one god or several?" he would not have objected.' In order to hide his disgust, and in an attempt to regain composure, he takes refuge momentarily in one of the Marabar caves. Adela ventures alone into a neighbouring cave and suffers an experience that is to change both of their lives for ever.

Friendship

The book begins with Dr Aziz entering into a discussion between his two barrister friends Hamidullah and Mahmoud Ali. 'Can the British and Indians be friends?' is the question that is being debated; when asked his opinion Dr Aziz tactfully declines to offer one, instead questioning the very merits of the debate: 'Why talk about the English? Brrrr … ! Why be either friends with the fellows or not friends?'

This question clearly troubled Forster a great deal, possibly explaining why it took him over a decade to conclude the book. In the final, deeply moving scene of this memorable work, Dr Aziz and his confidant Fielding ride together and, as they part company forever, Aziz declares those famous lines with which John chooses to close his account. And in support of Dr Aziz's contradictory conclusions, the animate and inanimate world around him echo in unison 'No, not yet', while the metaphysical world, signified by the sky, notes, 'No, not there.'

If friendship proved impossible 'then' and 'there', how might Forster view the chances of friendship between the British and Asian Muslims 'now' and 'here' in twenty-first-century pluralist Britain?

Crystal ball-gazing is a somewhat foolhardy activity, particularly so when one attempts to read the mind of the deceased who, in life, subscribed to a world view very different from one's own. Yet in spite of these cautionary notes, having had the opportunity to read about Forster's life from a number of sources, and being aware of his humanist beliefs, I am confident that he would have approved of many of the changes that have taken place since the publication of *A Passage to India*. The demise of the British Raj was, for example, a prophecy fulfilled. He would, I am sure, also have approved of pluralism per se, but unlike many contemporary social commentators would have noted that although abandoned as a political ideology, imperialism lives on in many more subtle guises. The large-scale migration to Britain that occurred throughout the latter half of the twentieth century from the euphemistically described New Commonwealth to meet labour shortages would, I believe, have been seen by Forster as one of the many manifestations of the new economic imperialism. He would also no doubt be aware that 'Macaulay syndrome' is far from eradicated and still has a central role in maintaining cultural imperialism. Eating cucumber sandwiches on the croquet lawn has, it seems, been a disproportionately common pastime for the Oxbridge-educated and Sandhurst-trained custodians of power of the ex-colonies.

If pressed on the question, I suspect that the response of this astute social critic would have been similar to that offered in *A Passage to India*. He would not, I suspect, have missed the damning MacPherson, Runnymede Trust and, most recently, King's Fund reports highlighting the issue of institutional discrimination faced by minority ethnic groups.[1-3] He would, I surmise, have suggested that for *genuine* friendship to blossom there is a need for both British and Asian people to come to terms with their own recent histories, and also, importantly, to understand far better the ethos and traditions of each other's world views. *'Only connect'* is Forster's enduring legacy, and in today's increasingly Internetted world, I suggest, this must be a goal for each and every one of us.[4]

References

1   MacPherson W (1999) *Report for the Stephen Lawrence Inquiry*. The Stationery Office, London.

2   Runnymede Trust (1997) *Islamophobia: a challenge for us all*. Runnymede Trust, London.

3   Coker N (2001) *Racism in Medicine*. King's Fund, London.

4   Sheikh A and Gatrad AR (2000) Breaking Barriers, Building Bridges. In: A Sheikh and AR Gatrad (eds) *Caring for Muslim Patients*. Radcliffe Medical Press, Oxford.

14

Mrs Dalloway

by Virginia Woolf (1925)

Wai-Ching Leung

Although *Mrs Dalloway* is only just over 200 pages long, I found it quite confusing when I read through it for the first time, although I thoroughly enjoyed it once I became familiar with it. I am used to novels written in the Victorian period by authors such as Charles Dickens and George Eliot, and they seem much easier to follow. The stories in these Victorian novels are mostly told by a third person who apparently knows everything from the outset. This third-person narrator even tells us what to think about each event and character. They are told largely in chronological order. Furthermore, there are usually predictable storylines or plots, which are resolved towards the end of the novel. For example, the protagonist usually becomes morally wiser as the novel progresses. The neat conclusion in these novels adds to the readers' satisfaction.

However, the absence of any of these features in *Mrs Dalloway* might initially make it rather confusing for the reader. First, most of the novel directly records the internal thoughts and consciousness of the characters. In this respect, Virginia Woolf was to some extent influenced by the 'stream of consciousness' style of another modernist novel, *Ulysses*, published by James Joyce in 1922. In

Ulysses, James Joyce included extended passages containing every thought of the characters, even if it is not relevant to the plot and appears incoherent to the reader. In *Mrs Dalloway*, Virginia Woolf adopted a less extreme form of this style. Instead of presenting to us every thought of each character, she selected the relevant internal thoughts for us to focus on. This is one reason why *Mrs Dalloway* is much shorter than *Ulysses*. There are moments when we get an impression that there is an external storyteller talking to us, although this is often mixed in with the internal thoughts of the character, and we are left with the task of sorting them out. Furthermore, the novel sometimes records the internal thoughts of one character at one moment and suddenly switches to those of another character without any warning. We must watch out for these changes of points of view in order to follow the novel. As a result, the sentences often appear long and fragmented. A good example is the following passage, right at the beginning of the novel, when we know very little about the protagonist, Mrs Clarissa Dalloway. It illustrates how the internal thoughts of an observer of Clarissa are mixed with the voice of an external storyteller:

> *For having lived in Westminster – how many years now? Over twenty, – one feels even in the midst of the traffic, or waking at night, Clarissa was positive, a particular hush, or solemnity; an indescribable pause; a suspense (but that might be her heart, affected, they said, by influenza) before Big Ben strikes. There! Out it boomed. (p 6)*

Second, the plot in *Mrs Dalloway* seems remarkably simple. The story takes place within a single day in familiar places in London such as Westminster, Piccadilly and Bond Street. The main protagonist is Mrs Clarissa Dalloway, a middle-aged, upper-middle-class woman who is married to Richard, an MP, and has recently convalesced from 'an illness'. The time is a single day in 1923, a few years after the First World War, when Clarissa is planning to hold an important party in the evening. The novel begins at 10am, marked clearly by Big Ben, when she leaves her home in Westminster to buy some flowers for the party. Around that part of London at the time are Septimus Warren Smith, a veteran of the

First World War, suffering from post-traumatic stress disorder associated with recurrent psychosis and depression, and his Italian wife, Rezia. The novel comprises essentially parallel descriptions of the experiences of Clarissa Dalloway and Septimus Smith during that one day. Clarissa is visited by her former lover, Peter Walsh, who has just returned from India. At the end of the novel, the evening party hosted by Clarissa Dalloway is attended by many upper-class people, including the Prime Minister. At the same time, Septimus Smith suffers a relapse of his psychosis. His wife, Rezia, desperately lacks support in looking after him in a foreign country. Both the general practitioner and the psychiatrist are unperceptive and unsympathetic. The visit by the general practitioner to take Septimus to a mental home results in Septimus's suicide while he is in a paranoid state of mind. The only connection between Clarissa's and the Smiths' experiences is that the psychiatrist brings the news of Septimus's death to the party, which deeply disturbs Clarissa. However, she determines not to let her own feelings spoil the atmosphere of the party.

Beneath this simple chronological narrative within a single day is a more complicated internal time of the characters. Their thoughts can suddenly move backwards as in a flashback, or move forwards as in a dream or wishful thinking. The author does not warn you of this shift from external to internal time and it makes it significantly more difficult for the reader to follow.

Third, we know the characters of the novel mainly through the thoughts of other characters. Unlike the Victorian novelists, the author does not give her own opinions about the characters themselves. Furthermore, the characters do not behave predictably.

Virginia Woolf, like many other modern novelists and painters, was influenced by the work of Sigmund Freud and other psychoanalysts. They highlighted the complexities of the human mind and personality, and suggested that people cannot be understood completely by an external observer. In one of Virginia Woolf's essays, she explained clearly why she wrote novels in the way she did:

Examine a moment an ordinary mind on an ordinary day. The mind receives a myriad impressions .... From all sides they come, an incessant shower of innumerable atoms; and as they fall, as they shape themselves into the life of Monday or Tuesday, the accent falls differently from of old .... Life is not a series of gig lamps symmetrically arranged; life is a luminous halo .... Is it not the task of the novelist to convey this varying, this unknown and uncircumscribed spirit, whatever aberration or complexity it may display, with as little mixture of the alien and external as possible? ... Let us record the atoms as they fall upon the mind in the order in which they fall, let us trace the pattern, however disconnected and incoherent in appearance, which each sight or incident scores upon the consciousness.[1]

This was precisely what she did in *Mrs Dalloway* – 'to record the atoms as they fall upon the minds' of each character. Once we get the gist of the novel, we can get very close to the private thoughts of each character and their impressions of one another.

Who was Virginia Woolf?

While it is important to know the author in reading any works of literature, it is perhaps much more so in *Mrs Dalloway*. The characters Clarissa Dalloway and Septimus Smith were based on aspects of Virginia Woolf herself. Many other characters were based on Virginia's friends and relatives. Much of the experience of these two characters was closely related to Virginia's own experience.

Virginia was born in 1882 at Hyde Park Gate, London, close to the setting for *Mrs Dalloway*. Both Virginia's mother (Julia Duckworth) and her father (Sir Leslie Stephen) had been married before. Virginia was the third child of this marriage. One of her half-sisters (from her father's side), like Virginia later, suffered from psychosis. Virginia's parents both came from upper-middle-class families and were well educated. Her father was a much-respected intellectual and a well-known literary critic. However, although her father and her two brothers, Thoby and Adrian, were educated at Cambridge, Virginia was mostly self-taught, as university education was almost closed to women at the time.

When Virginia was 13 years old, her mother died. This precipitated Virginia's first episode of psychosis, an illness which recurred throughout her life. Three further deaths, of her half-sister, her brother and her father, occurred within the next nine years. Virginia and her siblings became very lonely; they moved to a house at Gordon Square, Bloomsbury, where Septimus in *Mrs Dalloway* lived. Here, a group of friends of Virginia's brothers from Cambridge formed the Bloomsbury group, which advocated a new style of literary works different from that of the Victorians. This group at first provided Virginia with the education she lacked. However, it was clear from Virginia's work that she did not entirely approve of this group and was able to develop her own style of writing.

Virginia suffered from recurrences of her psychotic illness between 1910 and 1915, during which time she was admitted to Twickenham nursing home away from her family. This experience contributed to the vividness of her description of the psycho-pathology of those characters in her novels with mental illness, and her criticisms of doctors who insisted on patients being admitted against their will. The most significant event for Virginia was her marriage to Leonard Woolf in 1912, when she was 30 years old, which provided a great source of support and stability for Virginia to continue to write despite her recurrent psychotic illness. Leonard was Jewish. He was himself a novelist, but was an administrator in Ceylon when he met Virginia. Leonard decided to give up this career and live in England with Virginia, because he knew Virginia's mental health would suffer if she were to live abroad with him. Because of Leonard's concern for Virginia's mental health, they moved from central London to Richmond, a quieter area of London. To help Virginia in recovering after relapses, Leonard and Virginia set up a printing press called the Hogarth Press in 1917. The Hogarth Press published almost all of Virginia's novels and this gave her entire control over the process. She enjoyed a happy married life although she apparently had a distaste for the physical side of her relationship.

Virginia Woolf wrote nine novels. Her first novel, *The Voyage Out*, was published in 1915. With the exception of *Orlando* (1928), the pattern of each novel is similar. They all search for meaning in people's awareness. Rather than focus on conventional plots, the narrative moves from feelings of anxiety at the beginning, to transient moments of freedom and finally 'vision' from a new perspective towards the end. Her two most famous novels are her fourth, *Mrs Dalloway,* published in 1925, and her fifth, *To the Lighthouse* (1927). Both novels are based on aspects of her own life. There was instant success with *Mrs Dalloway* and Virginia's reputation soared in the 1930s.

Unfortunately, her comparative stability was shaken in the late 1930s by the possibility of another world war and the deaths of some of her personal friends and relatives. Although she had been free of her psychotic episodes since 1915, she relapsed in 1941 and lost insight into her illness. One morning in March, she committed suicide by drowning herself in a river after writing letters to her husband and her sister.

Mrs Dalloway

We have now done enough preparation to start reading the novel. It begins with Clarissa buying some flowers one morning for the party that evening. The air is fresh and calm. This reminds her of one morning many years ago when she was 18 years old and Peter Walsh was around. We are then led suddenly and directly into Clarissa's rumination about her past friendship with Peter. He still writes to her, but his letters are dull. He will come back from India soon. However, we are not told who Peter is. While Clarissa is deep in thought, she is watched by her neighbour, Scrope Purvis, who thinks that Clarissa is charming. Big Ben strikes. As Clarissa enters a park, she meets Hugh Whitbread, her old friend, and his wife, Evelyn. Hugh agrees to come to Clarissa's party. His upper-class culture makes Clarissa feel belittled. We are once more immersed in Clarissa's deep thoughts. Both her husband, Richard, and Peter Walsh dislike Hugh, as they think him incapable of sympathy for other people. Thinking of Peter, Clarissa cannot help reflecting that it would have been nice to walk with him on a morning like this. Peter would care about the state of the world. Memories rush to Clarissa's mind of her arguments with Peter that made her realise that she could not marry him because he would not give her any independence. Peter had retorted that

Clarissa was so concerned with superficialities that she would be a perfect hostess to the Prime Minister. Clarissa thinks she should buy a suitable book to give to Evelyn that evening. She questions her own motive for buying the book – so that she will be liked, rather than because of her own feeling for Evelyn. She wanders up Bond Street and reflects that, although she likes the delicate gloves she sees on sale there, her daughter, Elizabeth, is not at all interested in them. Instead, Elizabeth is friendly with Miss Kilman, a Christian evangelist who makes Clarissa feel small because of her faith and poverty. Clarissa hates Miss Kilman but cannot face the reality of her emotions, which have been like 'a monster' inside her since her recent illness.

Let us take stock of these first ten pages of the novel. You might find even this summary of events fragmented. Virginia Woolf introduces the various characters, both as they are encountered by Clarissa and as they naturally arise in her mind, almost by 'free association', within less than an hour. We come to know about Clarissa from what others think of her, and her own private thoughts. We learn about events that span several decades. Like Virginia herself, Clarissa resents male domination and has chosen a husband who will give her a degree of independence. While Clarissa thinks of Hugh Whitbread as an upper-class snob, she is herself considered in a similar light by her daughter, Elizabeth, and Peter. Clarissa's past illness and her struggle with her feelings recall Virginia's own experience. We are now prepared to meet Clarissa's 'double', Septimus Warren Smith, a sufferer from serious mental illness.

Septimus Smith – Clarissa's double

While Clarissa is in the flower shop, she hears a 'violent explosion' from a car outside. Passers-by get very excited and stay to watch. There are rumours that the car belongs to the Queen, the Prince of Wales or the Prime Minister. The street is so congested that Septimus Warren Smith, a 30-year-old veteran of the First World War who suffers from post-traumatic stress disorder, cannot pass through. He is clearly paranoid and has delusions of reference.

And there the motor car stood, with drawn blinds, and upon them a curious pattern like a tree, Septimus thought, and this gradual draw-ing together of everything to one centre before his eyes, terrified him, ... as if some horror had come almost to the surface and was about to burst into flames. The world wavered and quivered and threatened to burst into flames. It is I who am blocking the way, he thought. Was he not being looked at and pointed at; was he not weighted there, rooted to the pavement, for a purpose? But for what purpose? (p 18)

His Italian wife, Rezia, becomes very embarrassed. She imagines that the crowd must have noticed his strange behaviour, especially as he has threatened to kill himself. On the other hand, Clarissa hopes that the car belongs to the Queen and that her association with this level of society will give her greater importance at the party. When the car has moved on, a crowd gathers outside Buckingham Palace trying to decipher the advertisement written across the sky by an aeroplane. As their general practitioner, Dr Holmes, has previously suggested to Rezia that she should distract Septimus if he becomes ill again, she tries to draw his attention to the letters. However, this merely induces delusional perception and delusion of reference, which Septimus becomes totally engrossed in.

So, thought Septimus, looking up, they are signalling to me ... this beauty, this exquisite beauty, and tears filled his eyes as he looked at the smoke words languishing and melting in the sky and bestowing upon him, in their inexhaustible charity and laughing goodness one shape after another of unimaginable beauty and signalling their intention to provide him, for nothing, for ever, for looking merely, with beauty, more beauty! (p 25)

Rezia feels extremely anxious and isolated. She is very surprised that Dr Holmes has told her there was nothing wrong with him, when she knows he has been very ill. It is clear that, based on her own experience, Virginia Woolf did not think highly of doctors at the time. A young girl from Edinburgh visiting London for the first time asks Rezia for directions to the underground station. Rezia is anxious to ensure that she does not notice Septimus's mental illness, and replies abruptly. The young girl is seriously disturbed. She is terrified by Septimus.

Both seemed queer, [she] thought. Everything seemed very queer ... the young woman seeming foreign, the man looking queer; so that should she be very old she would still remember ... and the man – he seemed awfully odd; quarrelling, perhaps; parting for ever, perhaps; something was up, she knew. (p 30)

Virginia Woolf illustrates how mental health patients can acquire long-term stigma, as well as showing the enormous difficulties relatives of mental health patients face in caring for them.

Continuing the story of Mrs Dalloway: the surprise reappearance of Peter

Virginia has now introduced us to both protagonists, Clarissa and Septimus Smith. Although they are briefly in the same place in London, they have not exactly met or communicated with each other. Nor do their worlds meet until Clarissa hears of Septimus's death 16 hours later, at the end of the novel. Symbolically, however, the two characters are very closely related. Perhaps Septimus has the darker aspects of Clarissa's personality, which she would rather not acknowledge to herself. We might think of Septimus as Clarissa's alter ego.

We are now led through the experience of both characters in parallel. Clarissa returns home and goes upstairs to the attic room that she has occupied since her 'illness'. We are not told precisely what illness she had, although there is a reference early on to her heart being affected by 'influenza' (perhaps a Coxsackie virus). It is possible to take this at face value, but I would favour a metaphorical interpretation of the idea of 'heart trouble' to suggest a psychological illness. There is a clear correspondence between what goes on in Clarissa's mind and in that of Septimus Smith. For example, we can judge from Clarissa's internal thoughts that she has wild mood swings and makes associations between unrelated ideas. Clarissa is different from Septimus in that she can contain these ideas inside her head without their disturbing her behaviour. As we noted above, Clarissa has great difficulty in facing her own negative feelings towards other people such as Mrs Kilman, which points to an emotional rather than a physical origin of Clarissa's illness. When Virginia Woolf first conceived Mrs Dalloway, she intended the central character to commit suicide. Although she spared her heroine by inventing Septimus Smith, Clarissa remains an emotionally fragile person. Now let us return to the story.

Clarissa clearly has an inner conflict. On the one hand, she needs privacy to maintain her full sense of identity, as Virginia herself did. On the other hand, she is looking forward to acting as hostess at the evening party. We are once more drawn into Clarissa's memory when she was young. She remembers fondly her passionate friendship with Sally Seton, how she enjoyed the kiss Sally gave her, and their resentment of the intrusion by Peter Walsh. Thinking of Peter, she wonders whether he will see her as older when he returns from India, as she has become quite pale with her illness. At that moment, the doorbell rings and it is Peter himself. They have an emotional reunion. Peter thinks that Clarissa looks older and Clarissa thinks Peter is exactly the same as he was. As they remember the past, Peter becomes upset about Clarissa's refusal to marry him, while Clarissa is immersed in her own memory. He shows contempt for her upper-class values, but at the same time acknowledges that he has less control than she has over both material and spiritual achievements. Peter confronts Clarissa by asking her whether she has been really happy with her husband, Richard. In her own thoughts, Clarissa reflects that her life might have been less restricted if she had married Peter, but she would not have been able to tolerate Peter's intrusion into her life. Before Clarissa can answer Peter's question directly, her daughter, Elizabeth, arrives. Peter becomes embarrassed and leaves Clarissa's home immediately and Clarissa reminds him to come to the party that evening.

Here, we are invited into the internal thoughts of both Clarissa and Peter. There is clearly an emotional attachment between them. There are also clear contrasts between Clarissa's upper-class values and Peter's socialist beliefs, as well as Clarissa's need for privacy and Peter's habit of intrusion into it. We are also reminded of the contrast between Septimus's vulnerability and how Clarissa in her mental illness was protected by her upper-class background.

Transition to the world of Septimus Smith: Peter's dream

Virginia Woolf makes use of Peter to bring us back to the world of Septimus Smith. Peter leaves Clarissa's house as Big Ben is striking 11.30am. We are immersed once more in Peter's memories of being refused marriage by Clarissa, and her recent mental illness reminds Peter of the inevitability of death. Peter falls asleep on a bench beside a nurse, who is knitting, and we also share his dreams. In his dream, a solitary traveller sees a great ride and a giant female figure at the end of the path. The solitary traveller rides and reaches the female figure. Peter is comforted but does not know whom to reply to. Suddenly Peter wakes up, exclaiming, 'The death of the soul'. According to Freud's theory, dreams are our means of experiencing what we wish for in our unconscious (i.e. wish fulfilment). As these wishes often arouse anxieties, we are prevented from becoming conscious of them by the psychological mechanism of 'repression'. Instead, these wishes emerge in heavily disguised forms in our dreams. The solitary traveller clearly represents Peter himself. We might speculate that Peter lacks self-esteem and feels threatened by women. We might also think that Peter longs for spiritual support. Peter then remembers a scene one morning many years ago when he disagreed with Clarissa's opinion that it was improper to be pregnant before marriage. As the day passed, they sulked. At supper, he noticed that Clarissa was speaking to a conventional young man, Richard Dalloway, who held upper-class values. Peter 'knew' immediately that Richard would marry Clarissa. Peter became emotional and asked ridiculous and demanding questions of Clarissa. Their relationship ended that night. This past episode is crucial to Clarissa's decision to marry Richard instead of Peter. We might speculate that marriage with Richard instead of Peter might have been better in preventing a relapse of Clarissa's illness, in the same way that marriage with Leonard Woolf protected Virginia against recurrence of her mental illness for some time. Peter begins to take notice of the external world. The child who is being looked after by the nurse runs into the leg of Rezia Smith. We are brought again to the worlds of Rezia and Septimus Smith.

Continuing with the story of Septimus Smith

Rezia ruminates about her lack of support in looking after Septimus in London, resents Dr Holmes's failure to recognise her husband's illness and thinks about going back to Italy. She reaches out to Septimus but he notices that she is not wearing her wedding ring. Rezia explains that her fingers have grown so thin that it no longer fits. This explanation induces another set of paranoid and somewhat grandiose delusions in Septimus:

> *The marriage was over, he thought, with agony, with relief. The rope was cut; he mounted; he was free, and it was decreed that he, Septimus, the lord of men, should be free; alone (since his wife had thrown away her wedding ring; since she had left him), he, Septimus, was alone, called forth in advance of the mass of men to hear the truth, to learn the meaning, which now at last, after all the toils of civilisation – Greeks, Romans, Shakespeare, Darwin, and now himself – was to be given whole to .... (p 75)*

Rezia tells him that it is 'time to go', but the word 'time' triggers yet further hallucinations and delusions. Septimus hears the voice of his friend Evans, who was killed in Thessaly during the First World War:

> *The word 'time' split its husk ... an immortal ode to Time. He sang. Evans answered from behind the tree. The dead were in Thessaly, Evans sang, among the orchids. There they waited till the War was over, and now the dead, now Evans himself –*
> *'For God's sake don't come!' Septimus cried out. For he could not look upon the dead.*
> *But the branches parted. A man in grey was actually walking towards them. It was Evans! But no mud was on him; no wounds; he was not changed. (p 78)*

His feelings have been numbed after his experience in the First World War. Although he married Rezia in Italy with the hope that she might be able to restore his feelings, it has not worked: Rezia cannot communicate with him.

General practitioners, psychiatrists and mental health 'sections'

Virginia Woolf now shows us how the medical profession sometimes fails patients with mental illness. Rezia and Septimus return to their flat in Bloomsbury. Septimus wonders whether he will go mad and finally agrees for a doctor to be called. Dr Holmes, a general practitioner, visits. He is judgemental and decides there is nothing physically wrong with Septimus, only his 'crimes' during the War. He prescribes a little bromide, a mild sedative.

> There was nothing whatever the matter, said Dr Holmes. ... So there was no excuse; nothing whatever the matter, except the sin for which human nature had condemned him to death; that he did not feel. He had not cared when Evans was killed; that was worst; but all the other crimes raised their heads and shook their fingers and jeered and sneered over the rail of the bed in the early hours of the morning at the prostrate body which lay realising its degradation; how he had married his wife without loving her; had lied to her; seduced her .... The verdict of human nature on such a wretch was death. (pp 100–1)

He visits again but again pronounces that 'health is largely a matter in our own control' and advises Septimus to 'throw yourself into outside interests; take some hobby'. The next time Holmes calls, Septimus refuses to see him and talks about suicide. Holmes pushes past Rezia and continues to be judgemental.

> So you are in a funk ... didn't [talking about suicide] give [your wife] a very odd idea of English husbands? Didn't one owe perhaps a duty to one's wife? Wouldn't it be better to do something instead of lying in bed? (p 102)

Septimus reacts very badly and his hallucinations and delusions become more marked. He considers Dr Holmes as representative of the evil of human nature, and when he thinks he can hear his dead friend Evans talking from behind a screen, Rezia calls Dr Holmes in a panic, but Septimus screams 'you brute' as he approaches. Dr Holmes's authoritarian attitude is shown by his comment 'now what's all this about, talking nonsense to frighten your wife?' Dr Holmes also becomes annoyed and advises Rezia to take Septimus to see a Harley Street psychiatrist, Sir William Bradshaw.

The psychiatrist has excellent diagnostic acumen and makes a diagnosis of 'complete physical and nervous breakdown' as Septimus walks through the door. He takes a careful history, carries out a mental state examination and elicits the presence of serious suicidal ideation. He advises Septimus to be admitted to a psychiatric home away from Rezia – 'it was merely a question of rest, of rest, rest, rest; a long rest in bed' – but Septimus refuses. Sir William prescribes a sedative and explains to Rezia that he will have to apply for the appropriate mental health certification that evening as the patient is suicidal. Septimus asks whether Sir William would let him go if he confesses his crimes, but he cannot think of any crimes he has committed. Rezia does not consider Sir William 'a nice man' because he has given them only 45 minutes of his time before making such an important decision for them. Unusually, Virginia Woolf interjects directly, probably from her own experience that, rather than healing patients, Sir William's action might be seen as an attempt to convert and mould patients into an unoriginal form that the doctor prefers. In effect, he takes the life out of his patients.

Back in his flat, Septimus becomes agitated, hallucinates and has delusions. Rezia is distrustful of Sir William and promises Septimus that she will not let him be taken away by force to the psychiatric home. Septimus is pleased that Rezia can at last 'defeat both Holmes and Bradshaw'. When Dr Holmes arrives to take Septimus to the psychiatric home, Rezia tries to stop him seeing Septimus. However, he pushes past Rezia, and Septimus can hear him coming upstairs. Septimus is determined that neither Holmes nor Bradshaw will 'get him'. He looks around, but the bread knife, the gas fire and the razor are either unavailable or unsuitable tools at the time, so the option left is 'the tiresome, the troublesome and rather melodramatic business of opening the window and throwing himself out'. To Septimus, 'it is their (Holmes's and Bradshaw's) idea of tragedy, not his or Rezia's. Holmes and Bradshaw liked that sort of thing.' He sits on the sill and waits until the last moment because 'he did not want to die.

Life was too good.' However, when he sees Holmes at the door, he cries 'I'll give it you!' and throws himself out of the window.

Virginia Woolf mocks Dr Holmes's lack of empathy and humanity. He cries 'the coward!' as he enters Septimus's room. His reaction after the event is particularly illuminating: 'Who could have foretold it? A sudden impulse, no one was in the least to blame (he told Mrs Filmer). And why the devil he did it, Dr Holmes could not conceive' (p 165).

You might like to reflect for a moment on how you could have avoided this tragedy if you and your social worker colleague had to put a patient on section 4 of the Mental Health Act under such a situation.

Your turn

We have now gone through more than half of the novel. We are now taken back to the story of Clarissa up until the end of the evening party, when most of the characters in the novel meet. The Prime Minister also attends the party.

Now it is your turn to read Clarissa's and Peter's thoughts about each other, what happens at the party and what the Prime Minister is like. Has Clarissa actually been happy with her husband, Richard, and her daughter, Elizabeth? Was she wise to refuse Peter? What happened to Sally Seton? Why are the experiences of the two sufferers from illness, Clarissa and Septimus, so different? More significantly, how will Clarissa react to the news of Septimus's death? If you have recent psychiatric experience, you might like to analyse the detailed psychopathological descriptions of both protagonists. Last but not least, how is Virginia Woolf's own life experience reflected in this novel? If you think about these issues carefully, you will find the messages in this novel much deeper and richer than they initially appear and you will begin to enjoy the novel.

The text

Mrs Dalloway by Virginia Woolf was first published in 1925. I used the edition published by Penguin Popular Classics in 1996. (All page references in this chapter are to the Penguin edition.)

Reference

1   Woolf V (1925) Modern fiction. In: *The Common Reader*. Hogarth Press, London. The essay is also contained in: Woolf V (1967) *Collected Essays*, vol 11. Chatto and Windus, London.

Extracts from both books reproduced by kind permission of the Society of Authors as the literary representative of the estate of Virginia Woolf.

15

Decline and Fall

by Evelyn Waugh (1928)

I discovered *Decline and Fall* when I was a student and I thought it was the funniest book ever written. I must have read it a dozen times (it's quite short) and while enjoying it, I would frequently roll about laughing and insist on reading bits out to anyone who would listen. However, until I decided to write about it, I hadn't taken it off the shelf for many years. And when I started reading it again, I was surprised to find that parts of it made me feel quite uncomfortable. Much of it I still found hilarious and it is brilliantly written; but there is no doubt that a lot of the jokes now seem horribly racist in character. Of course, I knew that Evelyn Waugh's politics were well to the right of the *Daily Telegraph,* but my previous impression had been that the humour and the elegance of the writing placed it somehow outside politics. But times have changed since my student days, and a lot of the casual insults to people unfortunate enough not to be of Anglo-Saxon or Norman descent are just no longer acceptable. Instead of making us laugh, they just make us squirm with embarrassment. So, is this established classic and favourite book of my student self no longer suitable reading for impressionable young people? Published in 1928, it was Evelyn Waugh's first novel and I wondered if some of his later ones, like the equally hilarious (some would say even funnier) *Scoop*, about the world of journalism, were less tainted by racism. Or what about *Brideshead Revisited*, serialised for family viewing by the BBC? Alas, a quick flip through both books soon turned up the same racist attitudes and embarrassing mockery of non-whites.

What should I do? I really wanted to share with you some of the classic scenes from a book which had meant so much to me. But *Decline and Fall* no longer seemed to be quite the same book. In the end I decided that we would go through it together, enjoy the parts that were still funny, take a hard look at the unsavoury passages and try to reach a judgement. Is Evelyn a brilliant satirist or a Waugh criminal? Can he be both? Let us begin.

Unfortunate incident at Oxford

The story opens with a Prelude. We are in the cosy, all-male, upper-class confines of an Oxford college in the 1920s. The junior dean and the domestic bursar, two rather timid dons, are sitting in a room overlooking the garden quadrangle, listening to the uproar coming from the Bollinger Club dinner, taking place two staircases away. The Bollingers are all aristocratic young men of impeccable breeding but little patience with culture, learning or the lower social orders. When they are drunk they can do a lot of damage. The two tutors (Mr Sniggs and Mr Postlethwaite) are hoping they will get very drunk and do plenty of damage because the ensuing fines will allow them to open a few bottles of vintage college port. They will not be disappointed. 'It'll be more if they attack the chapel,' says Mr Sniggs. 'Oh, please God, make them attack the chapel.'

Soon they hear what Evelyn Waugh famously describes as 'the sound of English county families baying for broken glass'. The Bollingers burst out into the quad in their bottle-green evening coats and set about smashing up the rooms of any fellow students known to be interested in studying or the arts. They wreck a grand piano, tear up a prize poem and throw a Matisse painting into a water jug.

Waugh then cuts to another part of the college and introduces us to his 'hero', Paul Pennyfeather. Paul is a totally different kind of undergraduate: he is mild, earnest, studious and upper middle class, rather than county. He is reading for the Church. He has moderate habits (he drinks exactly one and a half pints of beer a day and smokes a pipe); he is interested in the League of Nations and has a few earnest, hard-working friends like himself. Paul is one of the great innocents of English literature, who seem to stumble, unwittingly, into fantastic plots, which are not of their making and somehow emerge unscathed. Sometimes they end up a little wiser, but not always.

On the night of the Bollinger dinner, Paul is returning contentedly from a meeting of the League of Nations Society. He enters the college, puts away his bicycle, and – as he walks across the quad to his rooms – he is set upon and debagged (i.e. deprived of his trousers) by the upper-class rowdies. Mr Sniggs observes the scene and reassures his colleague that the person they have caught is 'someone of no importance'. The next morning the master of the college is informed that Paul was seen running the whole length of the quadrangle without his trousers. 'It is not the conduct we expect from a scholar,' says the master firmly, and poor, innocent Paul is expelled from the college for indecent behaviour. Meekly, he packs his bags and prepares to leave. On his way through the gate, he gives a farewell tip to the college porter who says: 'I expect you'll become a schoolmaster, sir. That's what most of the gentlemen does, sir, as gets sent down for indecent behaviour.' That line always used to make me laugh (it still does). But then I think about child abuse and paedophiles and I begin to think there may be a sinister truth wrapped up in the jest.

Part one: Paul becomes a schoolmaster

In the first chapter of Part One, we find that Paul has taken the porter's advice and gone to a 'scholastic agency' to try and find a teaching post. The agency in question is called Church and Gargoyle (I believe the real-life equivalent is called Gabbitas and Thring, which is nearly as good). The proprietor is a Mr Levy. Why Mr Levy? I wonder. Are we in for some snide anti-Semitism? No, Mr Levy is not in the least Jewish – the real racism comes later. Church and Gargoyle have an excellent classification system for our so-called public schools. They are graded as Leading

School, First-rate School, Good School and School. 'Frankly,' confides Mr Levy to Paul, 'School is pretty bad.' Those of you who are still anxiously looking for suitable schools for your children would, I'm sure, be only too grateful for such a useful grading system. The next day, Paul is interviewed by Dr Augustus Fagan Esq PhD for a vacant position at Llanabba Castle School in North Wales. Here is Waugh's description of the headmaster: 'He was very tall and very old and very well dressed; he had sunken eyes and rather long white hair over jet black eyebrows. His head was very long and swayed lightly as he spoke; his voice had a thousand modulations, as though at some time he had taken lessons in elocution; the backs of his hands were hairy and his fingers were crooked like claws.'

I found myself delighted all over again by the brilliance of Waugh's writing. He starts off his sketch of Fagan by suggesting a distinguished old scholar with a beautiful voice – then, right at the end, he hits you with the hairy, clawed hands and the doctor suddenly seems more like a werewolf. Dr Fagan dismisses Paul's lack of experience ('that is in many ways an advantage') and he is engaged for the position of junior assistant master at a salary of £90 a year.

I have now read two chapters and I'm really enjoying myself. I have had to leave out three-quarters of the funny lines because there simply isn't room for them. Practically every sentence is a perfect ace. The man is a genius and so far not really seriously fascist. But we've hardly begun. The rest of Part One is a sort of parody of the classic public school story, but unusually, as seen from the point of view of the staff rather than the boys. We meet Paul's two colleagues, both in their different ways, delightful characters. The first is 'Captain' Grimes, a short man of about 30 (I always thought of him as much older) with a bald head, a red moustache and a wooden leg. Grimes is a bit of a bounder and is always finding himself 'in the soup', as he calls it, as a result of a recurrent and unmentionable misdemeanour. Grimes is clearly disreputable, despite his Harrow education. The boys know he is not really a gentleman, but they have a grudging respect for him because he carries a big walking stick with which to beat them if they are cheeky. The other staff member at Llanabba is totally unable to maintain discipline. His name is Prendergast (or 'Prendy') and he is a nervous ex-clergyman who had to give up his cosy parish because of Doubts. ('I couldn't understand why God had made the world at all.')

Although Grimes and Prendy and Dr Fagan are caricatured, they have a Dickensian vitality and are quite believable; and even though Llanabba Castle is an improbable sort of school, its dark-panelled rooms and cooking smells make its presence powerful too; soon I feel that I am also sitting in the common room with Paul and his colleagues wondering if we will be able to slip out to the village pub after dinner. But I am running ahead a little. It is still Paul's first evening at Llanabba and Dr Fagan, wearing a velvet dinner jacket, is outlining his duties. Paul is to have the fifth form for the rest of the term and is also to be put in charge of the games, the carpentry class and the fire drill.

'And I forgot, do you teach music?'
'I'm afraid not.'
'Unfortunate, most unfortunate. I understood from Mr Levy that you did. I have arranged for you to take Beste-Chetwynde in organ lessons twice a week. Well, you must do the best you can. There goes the bell for dinner. I won't detain you.'

Before dismissing Paul the doctor adds a warning not to tell the boys the reason for his leaving Oxford prematurely. 'We schoolmasters must temper discretion with deceit.' Fortunately, Beste-Chetwynde proves to be an amiable young man who doesn't mind in the least that his organ teacher is totally ignorant of music.

After dinner, Grimes takes Paul off to the pub and starts to tell him his troubles. Not the least of these is his engagement to Flossie, the elder of the doctor's two daughters. This, he sees as a kind of insurance policy against the next time he finds himself 'in the soup'. This seems to happen to Grimes about every six weeks. It has something to do with temperament and something to do with sex. However, he has always been saved from disaster by the fact that he is a public school man. '"There's a blessed equity in the English social system," said Grimes, "that ensures the public-school man against starvation. One goes through four or five years of perfect hell at an age when life is bound to be hell, anyway, and, after that, the social system never lets one down."' Grimes relates some of his previous escapes from a watery death in the soup and the two schoolmasters have a pleasant evening together. Towards the end, Philbrick, the school butler, appears and asks if either of them would like an introduction to a young lady. They send him packing and Grimes says that, for him, 'Women are an enigma.' When I first read *Decline and Fall*, I assumed, in my innocence, that Grimes's sexual misdemeanours involved enigmatic but grown-up women. Now I am painfully aware that he is a serial child abuser and that Waugh thought this was amusing.

First day in the classroom

The following morning Paul has to face the fifth form for the first time. 'But what am I to teach them?' he asks Grimes in a panic. Grimes's advice is not to try and teach them anything to begin with. Just to keep them quiet. 'Now that's something I've never learned to do', says poor Mr Prendergast.

The following scene in the classroom is quite wonderful. People who have read it never forget it and will happily quote it to you word for word. 'Ten boys sat before him, their hands folded, their eyes bright with expectation.' The first one says 'Good morning, sir', and Paul says 'Good morning' back. The next boy repeats the greeting and Paul again returns it, but when a third boy says 'Good morning' he suspects they are pulling his leg and tells him to shut up. 'At this, the boy took out a handkerchief and began to cry quietly. "Oh, sir," came a chorus of reproach, "you've hurt his feelings. He's very sensitive; it's his Welsh blood, you know."' Things have begun badly, just as Paul feared. He decides to try and re-establish control by finding out their names. The first boy says his name is Tangent, but the next one says his name is Tangent too:

'But you can't both be called Tangent.'
'No sir, I'm Tangent. He's just trying to be funny.'

When a third pupil claims the name too, Paul, in desperation, asks if there's anyone who isn't Tangent? Four or five others immediately protest that they wouldn't be called Tangent on the end of a barge pole. Soon the room is divided into those who are Tangent and those who aren't. A fight is beginning to break out between the two factions when Captain Grimes walks in and offers Paul his big walking stick to maintain discipline. (I don't know if your schooldays were anything like this; mine certainly were – but then I went to a very distinguished northern grammar school in the 1950s.) Clutching the big stick, Paul recovers his courage. He declares that he doesn't care a damn what any of them are called but, if there's another word from any of them, he will keep them in all afternoon. When Clutterbuck says this is impossible ('I'm going for a walk with Captain Grimes'), Paul replies: 'then I shall very nearly kill you with this stick. Meanwhile, you will all write an essay on "Self-indulgence". There will be a prize of half a crown for the longest essay, irrespective of any possible merit.' When the bell rings, Clutterbuck has covered 16 pages and wins the prize.

> *'Did you find those boys difficult to manage?' asks Mr Prendergast, later.*
> *'Not at all,' said Paul.*

Sports day

The next few chapters are devoted to the planning and execution of the Annual School Sports ('unfortunately postponed last year, owing to the General Strike'). Paul, now described to the assembled school by Dr Fagan as 'a distinguished athlete', is put in charge of the arrangements. As far as the doctor is concerned, the only purpose of the sports is to provide an opportunity for him to impress the more rich and influential parents. He tells Paul that it's important to distribute the prizes evenly around the school; Beste-Chetwynde and 'little Lord Tangent' must each win an event as both their mothers are coming down specially. Tangent's mother is Lady Circumference; and Mrs Beste-Chetwynde is a society glamour queen with whom Paul is about to fall hopelessly in love. You might also like to know that her name is pronounced 'Beast-Cheating'.

On a rainy afternoon, Paul and Prendy tramp out to the playing fields with an assortment of boys and try to organise the heats. They are assisted by Philbrick, the butler, who tells Paul his life story. Paul is surprised to hear that Philbrick is not really a butler at all but a notorious master criminal. During the course of the book Philbrick tells each of the masters an entirely different version of his life story. When they finally confront him he says loftily that all the accounts are false, but one day, they will know his full story, 'which is stranger than any fiction'. Philbrick is a mysterious and slightly menacing character who pops up throughout the book in a variety of guises.

All too soon, Sports Day arrives and the school staff are in a frenzy of activity preparing for the visitors. There are some flowers and shrubs, and a large marquee where tea, sandwiches and champagne will be served. 'I am concerned with *style*,' says the doctor. 'I wish, for instance, we had a starting pistol.' Philbrick, the sinister butler, promptly offers a large service revolver, with which Tangent will later be accidentally shot in the foot by the hapless Mr Prendergast.

Here comes the racism

Now, so far, it has all been good clean, witty, satirical fun, hasn't it? But this is where the racism starts. Who are these strangers coming to join in the upper-class English entertainment? 'Ten men of revolting appearance were approaching from the drive. They were low of brow, crafty of eye and crooked of limb. They advanced huddled together with the loping tread of wolves .... They slavered at their mouths which hung loosely over their receding chins.'

They are the local stationmaster and his colleagues of the Llanabba Silver Band, who have been booked to play at the sports. They are, of course, Welsh, and they talk like comic music hall Taffies. Harmless enough, you may think, if not very original. But that description of their initial appearance, although marvellously written, makes me think, uncomfortably, of the Nazis and their racial stereotypes. And it gets worse: Dr Fagan seizes the opportunity to lecture Paul on the Welsh character, on which he has plans to write a monograph. 'From the earliest times, the Welsh have been looked on as an unclean people. It is thus that they have preserved their racial integrity. Their sons and daughters rarely mate with human-kind except their own blood relations.' Does that give you a bit of a shiver of recognition? Now it may be that Welsh people feel sufficiently secure these days to be able to laugh off that sort of nonsense. But substitute 'Jews' for 'Welsh' and then how does it read? Not funny at all.

The description of Sports Day is wonderful and I can safely leave you to read and enjoy it for yourselves. But I'd like you to rejoin me at the point where Mrs Beste-Chetwynde arrives in her silent, dove-grey limousine and steps out 'like the first breath of spring in the Champs-Élysées'. She is gorgeous, and as I told you, Paul falls in love with her. But she has brought a companion, a man called 'Chokey'. When Dr Fagan shakes hands with him, he is astonished to see that Chokey 'while graceful of bearing and irreproachably dressed, was coal black'. Waugh uses that line, intended apparently to give his readers a frisson of horror, to close the chapter.

Racism rampant

The next chapter (Chapter 9, The Sports – continued) is the most horribly racist of all. Chokey, whose full name is Sebastian Cholmondley, seems to bring out the worst kind of old-fashioned, imperialist, racist attitudes in everyone. It became fashionable, in the 1920s, for society hostesses to invite black American jazz musicians to their parties; some observers of the scene, including Waugh, were outraged. In this chapter, all the old prejudices and absurd stories of atrocities against the white man are produced with relish. The word 'nigger' is used repeatedly. Chokey defends himself vigorously and points out that he is a civilised and well-educated man. Far from being a pagan savage, he is an expert on ecclesiastical architecture. He pleads the cause of racial equality and even evokes echoes of *The Merchant of Venice* at one point. But, unlike Shylock, he has no chance of appearing as anything except an absurd racial caricature, a black buffoon, because Evelyn Waugh is writing his script. Although there are still many things in this chapter which make me laugh, on the whole I now find it makes me cringe with dismay and embarrassment. What can be done about it? I will return to these censorious thoughts a little later.

A couple of chapters later, Captain Grimes is in the soup again. He has appeared before Dr Fagan (in his role of Llanabba magistrate) and been convicted of an unnamed but undoubtedly pederastic offence. Grimes plays his trump card and reveals that he is engaged to the headmaster's daughter. This news upsets Dr Fagan considerably. 'He is not the son-in-law I should readily have chosen. I could have forgiven him his wooden leg, his slavish poverty, his moral turpitude and his abominable features ... if only he had been a *gentleman*.' He then goes on, hopefully, to offer Paul the post of son-in-law combined with a partnership in the school. Paul politely but firmly rejects this opportunity and he spends the evening in the pub commiserating with Grimes on the latter's forthcoming appointment with matrimony. In the end the reality of life as an intimate member of the doctor's household is too much for poor Grimes. He disappears and when a pile of his clothes appears on the beach it is assumed (wrongly) that the captain has decided to drown himself. On this note of mock solemnity, Part One of the book finishes.

Part Two: high society

In Part Two, our schooldays are over and there is a complete change of scene. We are translated to Margot Beste-Chetwynde's country seat at King's Thursday. The noble old house, which has been the home of the Earls of Pastmaster for centuries, has just been totally demolished and replaced by a chilly, aluminium and glass modernistic structure designed by a fashionable German architect, Professor Silenus. The professor believes that the creation of great art requires 'the elimination of the human element from the consideration of form'. This was a sly dig at the architect Le Corbusier, who had famously defined a house as 'a machine for living in'. Paul has been invited to tutor young Peter Beste-Chetwynde in the holidays. This gives him plenty of opportunities to talk to his pupil's lovely young mother and soon they are wandering hand in hand in the still beautifully landscaped grounds of King's Thursday. Margot can't bear to think of Paul going back to that awful school so she offers him a job helping her in the family business. She is rather vague about the nature of this enterprise but it seems to involve arranging jobs for young women in hotels, theatres and other places of entertainment in South America. At this stage, Paul is too innocent to see that the Pastmaster family make their money from what was then called white slave traffic and which we would call sex slavery or child abuse. There is a scene in which Paul helps Margot to interview some of the girls. He is surprised by her crisp, business-like attitude to her work and once again hears that lack of experience in an applicant for a job is an advantage. Is this supposed to be funny? Is it a savage attack on the involvement of the English upper classes in organised vice? Or is it some kind of metaphor for the moral degeneration of the once-admirable aristocracy? Before we have time to decide what to think, Paul is arrested on the morning of his intended wedding to Margot and charged with trafficking in prostitution. And thus, with a further decline and fall in Paul's fortunes, the second part of the novel ends.

Part Three: Paul in prison

Paul is convicted and sentenced to seven years, which is rather a shock. He is a little cross with Margot for allowing him to take the rap for her criminal activities; but he has to agree with her son, Peter, that the idea of the beautiful Margot in prison is totally unthinkable. Thanks to his social background, Paul adapts quite easily to prison life and is quite glad of the opportunity for quiet reflection. Before long, some of our old friends turn up again, for the worlds of public school, high society and penal servitude are closely interlinked. The first to put in an appearance is the sinister Philbrick, now a convict himself, and a highly regarded trusty. Then Mr Prendergast turns up as the new prison chaplain. Although he has apparently regained his faith, his new vocation seems to suit him little better than being a schoolmaster. An awful fate lies in store for Prendy, which I shall not reveal here, as I must leave you a few surprises. Later on, Paul is taken in hand by the prison governor, Sir Wilfred Lucas-Dockery, who, he learns, without surprise, is Philbrick's brother. Sir Wilfred is full of enthusiasm for penal reform and he decides to use Paul to try out some of his innovative and humane psychological ideas. These are, of course, ludicrous, and Waugh has some harmless right-wing fun at the expense of liberals and reformers. Meanwhile, in the world of Mayfair, Paul's plight has not been entirely forgotten by his old friends and beneficiaries. Margot arranges for him to have as many books as he wants, and portions of *pâté de foie gras* and other upper-class delicacies unaccountably appear on his prison food tray. On one occasion, an old burglar is accidentally given some caviar intended for Paul. He rejects it indignantly and has to be appeased with 'an unusually large lump of cold bacon'. The culture gap between the upper and the lower orders is always good for a joke with Evelyn, and I have to admit I was chuckling when I read about the burglar and his bacon.

What happens in the end, I shall let you find out for yourselves. I shall merely say that everything turns out very well for Paul and the world in which he really belongs is miraculously restored to him, thanks to his influential friends. Thanks also, perhaps, to 'Fortune, a much-maligned lady', in honour of whom the characters on two occasions drink a toast.

Reaching a verdict

Now it's time for us to weigh up the good and bad things about *Decline and Fall*. I have tried to share with you some of the joy and entertainment the book has given me since I first read it 40 years ago. I still think that it's a classic of English humour, with some wonderfully vibrant characters who are much more than caricatures. Some of the scenes, especially the school ones, have that special quality of remaining in your memory in clear detail. Evelyn Waugh's prose style is also quite delightful; clean, lucid, apparently simple, full of surprises. Every shot is delivered with perfect dead-pan aplomb. You will never catch even the flicker of a grin on the author's face. But was he also, in 1928, an angry young man? He clearly has the young fogey's aloof distaste for modernism and modernity, which he seems to associate with moral anarchy. But much of that satire has now lost its sting and what we remember is the wonderful black comedy. The real problem is that the book also contains examples of unpleasant racism, which are really not funny, and no longer acceptable in our more enlightened age. Can one excuse them on the grounds that they were written in 1928, when nearly everybody was racist to some degree? Should one see them in their historical context and not be such an oversensitive, whingeing liberal? No, that won't wash, because these passages (mainly in Chapter 9) give off an unpleasant smell that it's impossible for a liberal like me to ignore. On the other hand, we liberals don't approve of censorship and the suppression of books is not for us. So what is to be done? Should I advise people that *Decline and Fall* has forfeited its right to be considered a classic and should no longer be read by decent people, except as an example of decadent fascist literature?

No, that won't do either, because the rest of the book is too good to consign to oblivion. Waugh was a genius but a cranky, prejudiced, flawed genius. I think, if he were alive today, and I was his literary editor (very presumptuous, I know, but indulge me), I would advise him that modern editions of the book should omit most of Chapter 9 and some of the racism that glares out in other chapters. I think I would advise some modification of Captain Grimes's sexual preferences as well. David Bradshaw, in his introduction to the latest Penguin Classics edition (2001), does discuss the problem; he argues that when the racist passages are seen in context we can't take them seriously, because the prejudices are voiced by characters who are themselves morally debased. I have to disagree and I'd like to know what you think. So please read *Decline and Fall* as soon as you can. Prepare to be disturbed by Chapter 9, but enjoy the rest of the book, which contains some of the most brilliant and laughter-inducing writing of the twentieth century.

The text

Decline and Fall, first published by Chapman and Hall in 1928, is available in Penguin Modern Classics with an introduction by David Bradshaw. All material quoted from *Decline and Fall* by Evelyn Waugh (Copyright © Evelyn Waugh 1928) is reproduced by permission of PFD on behalf of the Evelyn Waugh Trust.

16

One Hundred Years of Solitude

by Gabriel García Márquez (1967)

In 1967 an amazing new novel exploded onto the literary scene. It was written by a young Colombian author and it soon became very popular, not just in Latin America but all over the world. Have you come across the phrase 'magical realism'? It was first used about this book, and although many other people have since tried to write in this style there is no substitute for the magic of the original. If you haven't read *One Hundred Years of Solitude*, it will now be my pleasure to introduce you to a story that will haunt your dreams. But first I'll introduce the author.

Gabriel García Márquez was born in a small town in Colombia in 1928 and he is still alive, so he must be about 75. He went to a Jesuit college in Bogotá and then escaped to Europe, where he became a journalist. His first book was published in 1947 and he soon became an established novelist. In *Leaf Storm*, in 1955, he introduced the fictional town of Macondo, which is also the setting for *One Hundred Years*. You may have read and enjoyed *Love in the Time of Cholera* (1985), which also has a touch of magic. But nothing in any of his other books really prepares you for the unique world of *One Hundred Years of Solitude*, which won Márquez the Nobel Prize for Literature in 1982.

Approaching the book

So what is *One Hundred Years of Solitude* all about? First of all, it's a family saga covering 100 years in the life of the Buendía family from maybe 1860 to 1960. If that seems vague, it's because we are not given any dates. Second, it is a sort of history of South America as seen through the experiences and imagination of the family and the community. And then there's the solitude. Macondo is an isolated community as we shall see, but most of the characters seem to have a way of shutting off their feelings and being unable to relate to other people. I have to admit that it's really rather a sad book, but it's also very funny and entertaining.

Chapter One

The family surname is Buendía, which I guess is a contraction of 'Buenos días', Spanish for 'Good day'. Opposite page one you will find a family tree. These are always helpful in family sagas and this one will be indispensable. However, it is a bit unusual in that all the men seem to be called Aureliano. No, that's not quite true, some of them are called José Arcadio. I suggest that you leave the genogram for the moment and read the unforgettable first sentences. After that I shall have difficulty in stopping you.

> *Many years later, as he faced the firing squad, Colonel Aureliano Buendía was to remember that distant afternoon when his father took him to discover ice. At that time Macondo was a village of twenty adobe houses, built on the bank of a river of clear water that ran along a bed of polished stones, which were white and enormous, like prehistoric eggs. The world was so recent that many things lacked names, and in order to indicate them it was necessary to point.*

So many ideas are introduced, so quickly, the effect is quite stunning. Before we have a chance to recover from the casual mention of the firing squad we are puzzling over the discovery of ice. We have to read on. We learn that the village of Macondo is regularly visited by a family of gypsies, led by the enigmatic Melquíades, who delights in showing the innocent villagers the world's wonders. Some of these are natural marvels such as magnets or lenses. However, we can't help noticing that Melquíades's magnet is powerful enough to draw pots and pans down from their shelves and make 'beams creak from the desperation of nails and screws trying to emerge'. Even long-lost objects emerged from their hiding places and 'were dragged along by Melquíades's magical irons. "Things have a life of their own," the gypsy proclaimed with a harsh accent. "It's simply a matter of waking up their souls."'

I think that gives you a good idea of what life in Macondo is going to be like. The real and the magical co-exist quite naturally and while people may be astonished they are not really surprised. In other words, we could be dreaming: but are we asleep or awake? On page two we are introduced to the first person on that family tree, the founder of Macondo, the patriarchal José Arcadio Buendía. JAB, as I shall call him, is fascinated by any kind of science or technology and gets totally absorbed in pushing ideas to their limits. He tries eagerly to use the magnets to drag up gold from the earth, although the honest Melquíades has warned him that this won't work. Then he tries to use the fire-producing power of the magnifying glass as a weapon of war. His sensible wife, Úrsula, is more concerned that he is going to set the house on fire. On a later visit, the gypsy provides him with some astronomical instruments. JAB shuts himself in a small room at the back of the house (the equivalent of the modern hobby-obsessed father's shed) for the entire rainy season and after much study and conjecture announces one day that: 'The earth is round like an orange.' At this point his wife loses her patience and smashes his astrolabe to the floor. The next gift from Melquíades is a complete alchemical laboratory with which JAB tries to double the quantity of the family's gold – without success.

This cornucopia of a first chapter continues with an account of the geographical explorations of JAB and his friends. Macondo seems to be entirely surrounded by swamps, but José Arcadio is convinced that it must be possible to find a route which will connect their little town with 'the great inventions'. The expedition sets off to the north where they come across a ghostly Spanish galleon, its ragged sails still hanging from its intact masts and inside it 'nothing but a thick forest of flowers'. Disappointingly, they soon reach the sea once again. When they return to Macondo, JAB wants to uproot the settlement and move it to somewhere more promising where, for example, there might be a magic liquid you could pour on the ground which would make the plants immediately bear fruit. But Úrsula firmly puts a stop to this nonsense by telling him she is not moving. 'Instead of going about worrying about your crazy inventions,' she tells him, 'you should be worrying about your sons.'

What about the children?

So it's time for us to take an interest in the children as well: the two boys and their sister occupy the second line of that rather strange family tree at the beginning. The boys are called José Arcadio (after his father) and Aureliano (after his father's obsession with gold). José Arcadio is 14, with a square head and thick hair. He is like his father but without his imagination. Aureliano (now aged 6) was the first child to be born in Macondo. 'He was silent and withdrawn and had wept in his mother's womb.' Oh dear. As we shall later learn, this is a bad sign, and the indication that a person will be incapable of love. This Aureliano, later to be Colonel Aureliano, will become perhaps the most solitary of all the self-absorbed members of the Buendía family: I don't accept that he is really incapable of love and evidence for this view will soon be placed before you. At any rate, he will inspire in all of us a good deal of affectionate concern. At the age of 3, Aureliano correctly predicts that a pot of soup, firmly placed on the table will suddenly tip over and spill. His mother is alarmed but when she tells his father he says that it is just 'a natural phenomenon'. That's the way things are in Macondo. As in dreams, whatever happens happens. However, JAB does start to take more interest in the boys' education. He invites them into his laboratory where he teaches them to read and write and do sums – and tells them about the wonders of the world. More gypsies come with dancing and music in the streets. They bring 'parrots painted all colours reciting Italian arias and a hen who laid a hundred golden eggs to the sound of a tambourine and a trained monkey who read minds and the multiple use machine that could be used at the same time to sew on buttons and reduce fevers ...'. By this time we are past protesting at the blurring of the line between physics and fantasy. This is Macondo and anything goes. This brilliant first chapter ends with the children being ushered into a tent to see the gypsies' most amazing novelty: an enormous transparent block full of coloured lights. The largest diamond in the world? No, it's a block of ice, 'the greatest invention of our time'. This is the moment that Aureliano will remember when he faces the firing squad.

The second chapter

I have to tell you now that although the book has 20 chapters of approximately equal length, they are neither named nor numbered. I have numbered them in my copy in pencil and to assist your navigation through the book, you may wish to do the same. Chapter 2 then, tells the back story of the founding of Macondo. It seems that José Arcadio and Úrsula are cousins, and when they marry she is terrified that if they have a child it will be born with the tail of a pig. (You may laugh but it had already happened once in the family, with tragic consequences.) So she equips herself with a massive pair of chastity pants. When her husband defeats a friend called Prudencio Aguilar in a cock-fight, Prudencio taunts him about his virility and so, unfortunately, JAB has to kill him. He holds Úrsula responsible for the death of his friend and orders her to take off her chastity pants before there are any more deaths. Prudencio comes back to haunt the couple (the dead get very lonely) and so they decide to leave town and found a new community far away across the mountains.

This chapter then picks up the story of the Buendías and their two sons in Macondo. José Arcadio (junior) develops a hormonal fascination with an earthy sex goddess called Pilar Ternera, who also tells fortunes. She provides the boy with a memorable sexual initiation (and remains on hand for 80 or so years to provide this service for young men of subsequent generations). Then the gypsies return with more wonders, including a magic carpet. Young José becomes infatuated with a thin young girl and runs off with the gypsies when they leave. He is not heard of again for some time. Meanwhile Úrsula has given birth to a daughter (Amaranta).

Chapter 3: the coming of Rebeca and the insomnia plague

As Chapter 3 begins, we find José Arcadio Buendía organising the planning and building of the town. He orders the freeing of the caged birds and their replacement with musical clocks so that the town is full of merry little tunes and synchronised chimes. Meanwhile Úrsula supports the family by making and selling little candied animals. Then a strange little girl called Rebeca arrives with a letter of introduction. She is 11 years old and her baggage consists of 'a small trunk, a little rocking chair with hand-painted flowers, and a canvas sack which kept making *clic-cloc* sounds where she carried her parents' bones'. At first Rebeca does not talk and she eats nothing but earth from the courtyard and whitewash off the walls. Úrsula manages to cure her of this habit (although she tends to revert to it during emotional crises). Unfortunately Rebeca has brought with her an infectious disease called the 'insomnia plague'. Soon nobody can sleep and at first it seems to be good fun, staying up all night. But they quickly discover that the insomnia plague also causes amnesia. People forget their own childhood and the identity of their friends. Eventually, even the names and purposes of everyday objects are forgotten. What is to be done? Aureliano (the younger son) comes up with the brilliant idea of labelling everything with its name and function before all recollection disappears. Tables and chairs and other household objects are all labelled as if in a museum. Even the cow has a sign round her neck saying *'This is the cow. She must be milked every morning.'* On the edge of the town they put up a sign saying MACONDO and another one on the main street that says GOD EXISTS. (I told you this strange book would make you laugh.) But why should insomnia cause dementia, I wondered. It seems to be something to do with being deprived of REM sleep and not being able to dream. If we can't dream we lose touch with our innermost selves (or souls?) and we become zombies. Or something like that.

You will be relieved to hear that the 'insomnia' doesn't last for ever. The folks of Macondo are cured by a magic drink provided by the mysterious old gypsy Melquíades, who turns up again just in time. The passage in which JAB recovers his memory and at the same time recognises his old friend is very moving. As usual, Melquíades has brought some more of the latest technology. This time it's the daguerrotype (an early kind of photographic process) and soon everyone is having their picture taken. JAB, with his obsessively enquiring mind, sets up cameras in different parts of the house to try and capture the image of God. Or, at least, to put an end once and for all to the controversy over His existence. As for Melquíades, he now moves in with the family and becomes increasingly inscrutable. He mutters to himself in a strange mixture of languages and spends a good deal of time scribbling undecipherable runes on pieces of crumbling parchment. I don't want you to forget those parchments because their meaning will one day come sharply into focus.

So many amazing things happen in this chapter, I haven't space to tell you them all. But the other major event is the arrival of the magistrate Don Apolinar Moscote and his family. It seems that the state has become aware of the existence of Macondo and has decided they need some law and order. JAB and the other leading citizens try to persuade him that he should pack his bags and go, but he refuses. So JAB picks him up by the lapels of his jacket, carries him down the main street and sets him down on his two feet on the swamp road. But he is back a week later escorted by 'six barefoot and ragged soldiers'. Eventually they come to an agreement: Don Apolinar is allowed to stay but without his soldiers. He is really quite a nice chap and everyone is charmed by his seven daughters. Especially Aureliano, who falls hopelessly in love with the youngest, aged nine. And about that we shall hear a good deal more.

Where do we go from here?

By this stage, I think you will be beginning to feel at home in Macondo and almost like a member of the Buendía family. You will have recovered from the shock of the insomnia plague, life has a dreamy holiday quality and there are some intriguing plot lines stretching ahead. In short, there is no need for me to take you through the rest of the book chapter by chapter. Instead, we shall have a longitudinal gaze at the lives of some of the main family members. I will also attempt to sketch an outline of the short history of Macondo and then attempt a summing up of the *One Hundred Years of Solitude* experience. Does that sound a good plan? Excellent.

José Arcadio Buendía and Úrsula

JAB is, of course, the founding father of the Buendías and his influence runs through the whole book. He can be a practical man when he wants to be (like when he is building a new town), but he is really much happier shut away in his alchemical laboratory working away at discovering the meaning of the universe. He is a gifted scientist: does he not work out from first principles and observation that 'the world is round like an orange'? But he is also a mystic and a believer in the supernatural. Well it's difficult to be anything else in Macondo: but Isaac Newton had similar tendencies and he lived in Cambridge. In fact, I've just realised that, for Newton and his fellow 'natural philosophers', Cambridge *was* a bit like Macondo – for them, alchemy and theology were just as important as mathematics for investigating the works of God. And, of course, Newton was a lover of solitude, just like JAB. In the end, poor José Arcadio Buendía slips off his bearings. He becomes obsessed with trying to use a pendulum as the source of energy for a flying machine. Unfortunately, he concludes, although a pendulum will lift anything, it is incapable of lifting itself. After the death of Melquíades he also begins to grieve bitterly for all the dead, including the man he killed and his own parents. Finally, in a fit of despair and rage, he seizes an iron bar and smashes up his laboratory and all his equipment. To prevent him from finishing off the house as well, they have to drag him out and tie him to the chestnut tree in the courtyard. And there he stays, for the rest of his life, poor fellow. The family feed him regularly and build him a shelter; Úrsula keeps him up to date with the news and various friendly ghosts keep dropping in to keep him company. But it's a heavy dose of solitude, all the same.

Úrsula, JAB's wife, is completely different. Her mission throughout her long life is to preserve the home and to keep the family functioning with some degree of normality. She is the one who looks after the children and grandchildren, sees to the housekeeping and home improvements, keeps family records, arranges marriages, supervises funerals and tries to get people to be less solitary. And, don't forget, she is often the only breadwinner with her successful trade in candy animals. At the end of the war, she tries to intervene with the revolutionary court to save the life of a decent ex-military governor by reminding the generals that she and the other mothers 'reserve the right to pull down your pants and give you a whipping at the first sign of disrespect'. Later on, she educates her great-great-grandson for the priesthood in the hope that he will avoid all the pitfalls that have brought about the downfall of previous Buendían men: war, fighting cocks, bad women and 'wild undertakings'. In Chapter 13, aged over 100, she starts to go blind, although because she knows the house and its inhabitants so well, it's a long time before anyone notices. In her blindness, she develops piercing and rather saddening insights about her children and their emotional isolation. In extreme old age she shrinks to the size of a child and is carried around the house and used as a plaything by the children, who think she is some kind of doll. She finally recovers her dignity and, before she dies, she embarks on a two-day-long prayer, which is a mixture of requests to God and bits of practical advice, such as how to stop the red ants from bringing the house down and never to let any Buendía marry a person of the same blood because their children will be born with the tail of a pig.

The second generation

The Buendías have two sons, José Arcadio and Aureliano, and a daughter, Amaranta (which means flower that never fades).

Colonel Aureliano Buendía

Aureliano, let me remind you, is the second son of JAB and Úrsula, and our story started with his recollection, as he was facing the firing squad, of the discovery of ice. Aureliano is the intellectual of the family who also becomes a famous soldier. He is also the most emotionally withdrawn. When he is not fighting in the revolutionary wars he likes to shut himself up in his workshop where he painstakingly manufactures little gold fish, applying one tiny golden scale at a time and finishing them off with little ruby eyes. Although he's not very sociable, I am fond of Aureliano and I think you will like him too. After he is suddenly smitten with love for Remedios, the magistrate's nine-year-old daughter, he becomes quite vulnerable for a while and writes her lots of love letters. Neither family is very keen on the match but eventually, when Remedios reaches puberty, they are married. Unhappily, the marriage is a brief one as Remedios is destined for an early death. The grieving Aureliano never recovers his capacity to love. He learns about politics while playing chess with his father-in-law and discovers the difference between Liberals and Conservatives. He decides he will be a Liberal and when war breaks out he leads a successful skirmish against the soldiers who have occupied Macondo and announces that from now on he is 'Colonel Aureliano Buendía'.

The revolutionary war rages on and off for nearly 20 years. We are told that 'Colonel Aureliano organized thirty-two armed uprisings and lost them all'. Nevertheless, he does seem to have some temporary successes and becomes a distinguished and respected figure. He survives the firing squad thanks to his brother, José Arcadio, who steps in with a loaded shotgun. Eventually he becomes disillusioned with the Liberals when their politicians ask him to tone down his revolutionary aims in order to 'broaden the popular support of the war'. This turns out to mean that there is really no difference between the Liberals and the Conservatives and 'all we are fighting for is power'. Aureliano, sickened by all the killing and the collapse of his idealism, negotiates the end of the war and deals quite brutally with those rebels who want to continue. He tries to commit suicide by shooting himself and fails.

Then he retires to his workshop and concentrates on handmaking those little gold fish, melting them down and remaking them for most of the rest of his life.

José Arcadio

José Arcadio (junior) is Aureliano's elder brother, and you may recall that at the end of Chapter 2 he ran off to join the gypsies. Well, he reappears suddenly in the fifth chapter, a huge young man, enormously strong and radiating masculine sexuality. All the women in Macondo go crazy for him and, I regret to say, he seems to make his living by gratifying their desires. However, he suddenly notices his adopted sister Rebeca (you know, that little girl who arrived carrying her parents' bones in a bag which goes *clic-cloc* and who also brought the insomnia/amnesia plague). 'You're a woman, little sister,' he tells her, and Rebeca succumbs instantly and passionately. So they get married, and young José Arcadio is next seen laying claim to lots of land that his father had previously given away. We have already seen that he intervenes fiercely to save his brother, the Colonel, from the firing squad. Shortly after that, for no obvious reason, he locks himself in the bathroom and shoots himself dead. A trickle of blood runs through the door, crosses the living room, goes out into the street, turns the corner and makes its way to Úrsula's kitchen to let the poor mother know what has happened. It's just typical of the way this family communicates. A systems therapist would probably be able to explain the whole thing. Or at least, would know the right questions to ask. I can't say I miss José Arcadio very much but I am very sad for his mother and of course his little sister-wife, Rebeca.

When the funeral is over, Rebeca shuts herself in her house and is not seen in the street again until many years later when she is a tiny old woman. Is this getting unbearable? It would be if it were not for the incomparable style which gives everything the distance and dream-like quality of a Greek myth. That, and Márquez's sense of humour.

Amaranta: the younger sister

There is a relatively light and lyrical period in the story (Chapter 4) when Amaranta and Rebeca are teenagers. Úrsula has just enlarged and beautified the family house. She imports all sorts of costly European furniture, curtains, carpets and tableware, and, most important of all, a pianola. For this is to be a very musical chapter. Along with the pianola comes Pietro Crespi, a fair-haired Italian young man with impeccable manners. He has been sent by the import house 'to assemble and tune the pianola, to instruct the purchasers in its functioning, and to teach them how to dance to the latest music printed on its six paper rolls'. Soon the new house is full of young people. There is music, there is dancing and there is love. Both Rebeca and Amaranta fall in love with the young Italian. When he goes away, Rebeca pines for him and writes him lots of love letters. Amaranta also writes a letter to Pietro but hides hers in her trunk. Úrsula finds herself having to care for two love-sick adolescent girls. Eventually Pietro and Rebeca get engaged and, by way of apology, Pietro offers to introduce Amaranta to his younger brother. Amaranta finds this totally humiliating. She gets very angry and her mother decides to send her away for a while. As she kisses Rebeca goodbye, Amaranta whispers in her ear: 'Don't get your hopes up. Even if they send me to the ends of the earth I'll find some way of stopping you getting married, even if I have to kill you.'

But, as we have seen, Rebeca's affection switches abruptly to José Arcadio junior, when that muscular, sensual young man returns from his travels. That would seem to leave the field clear for Amaranta to marry the disappointed Pietro Crespi. By this time he has set up a shop in Macondo and lives down the street from the Buendías. He and Amaranta have a very romantic courtship, encouraged by Úrsula, and all seems to be going wonderfully well. But, when Pietro names the wedding day, Amaranta tells him not to be so simple, and declares with a smile: 'I wouldn't marry you even if I were dead.' What has got into this strange girl? Is it slowly simmering revenge for his earlier preference for Rebeca? Tragedy follows and the music stops. Pietro cuts his wrists (another suicide) and Amaranta, in terrible remorse, puts her hand into the hot coals of the stove, giving herself a grievous burn. For the rest of her life she wears a black bandage of remorse on her hand and she too becomes a solitary. However, she does have a very sensual relationship with her nephew, a son of Colonel Aureliano. She allows him to see her naked throughout his childhood and even to come and play in her bed when he is an adolescent. There is much family concern about whether he should be allowed to marry his aunt. Their children will obviously have pigs' tails but young Aureliano says he doesn't care if they are armadillos. In the end, Amaranta turns him down too, and goes back to being a solitary, virginal spinster. Her last attempt to be sociable is at the end of her life when she generously offers to carry everyone's messages to the dead.

A brief look at the third and subsequent generations

You may be wondering, with all these suicides, and refusals of love, who is going to prevent the Buendía family from dying out. That responsibility rests with Arcadio, the illegitimate son of Pilar Ternera and José Arcadio junior. I haven't mentioned Arcadio so far for fear of confusing you. He is a rather shadowy, neglected boy who is brought up by his grandmother, Úrsula, but never really knows who his parents are. As if to compensate, he becomes the military governor of Macondo during the wars and is something of a tyrant. He marries an elusive and saintly woman called Santa Sofía de la Piedad (don't worry about the names, they are all in the family tree). They have three children. The eldest is a girl called Remedios the Beauty, who goes around the house innocently naked. Her beauty is so overwhelming that men die of love for her and one day she simply rises up to heaven and is seen no more. Remedios has twin brothers called, yes, I'm afraid so, Aureliano Segundo and José Arcadio Segundo. Aureliano 2 and José Arcadio 2 are supposed to have distinctive characters, following their prototypes, but I am never quite sure about the Segundo twins because they like muddling people about their identities, and it is possible that during their childhood they have permanently swapped names. In Chapter 13 there is a memorable eating contest in which Aureliano takes on a formidable but always graceful female adversary known as 'The Elephant'. There are many more wonderful episodes which I shall not have space to tell you about, but they are all there waiting for you, teeming and bubbling away in a book which is really not all that long. Aureliano is the father of the fourth generation (whose adventures I shall leave you to discover for yourselves) but it is his twin brother, José Arcadio Segundo, who passes on the obsessive interest in deciphering the manuscripts of Melquíades the gypsy. He teaches his little grand-nephew to read (his name? Would you believe – Aureliano?) and he is the one who finally discovers the meaning of the manu-scripts. I say discovers, but it takes a lot of hard work over several generations to read those parchments, an achievement of which the cryptographers of wartime Bletchley would have been very proud. We will return to the parchments before we close, but I haven't yet decided whether to reveal their secret to you.

A history of Macondo

I want now to leave the individual characters and trace the history of Macondo as a community. We know that it was originally settled as a primitive village by the founding families who crossed the mountains. José Arcadio Buendía, the paterfamilias, supervises the subsequent laying out of the town. After the insomnia plague, Macondo enjoys a brief period of complete independence before its existence comes to the notice of the authorities. Then the magistrate arrives and Macondo submits, unwillingly, to government. A priest arrives and the first church is built. Soon Macondo is involved in elections, which are clearly being rigged by the Government. There is an armed uprising leading, as we have seen, to nearly 20 years of revolutionary war. But which historical war did the author have in mind? We are never quite sure what period of history we are living through during our hundred-year stay in Macondo. Of course, it could be a conflation of all the wars of the nineteenth and twentieth centuries, but my guess is that Márquez is mainly thinking of the period from 1948 to the early

1960s, which he lived through himself, and which the Colombians call *La Violencia*. This, according to my historical researches on the Internet, was a time of recurrent guerrilla warfare, which was finally resolved by the formation of a coalition government. In other words, all the vested interests decided to combine to enforce peace and protect their property. No wonder Colonel Aureliano was disillusioned.

In the second half of the book, the twentieth century begins to intrude relentlessly on the solitude of Macondo. The railway arrives ('something frightful', as one woman describes it, 'like a kitchen dragging a village behind it'.). Next to come are electricity and the cinema, both of which delight and puzzle the citizens. But capitalism and exploitation are not far behind. Businessmen from North America ('gringos') appear in the town to nose out the possibilities of large-scale banana growing. On the other side of the railway line, they establish a town of their own, surrounded by an electrified fence. The old town fills up with whores, drunks and adventurers, who build their houses on vacant lots without permission. The barefoot policemen are replaced by hired assassins. Macondo is no longer the pleasant (if bizarre) little backwater it used to be. It has become overcrowded, noisy and dangerous. Was this the fate of numerous little South American towns? I wouldn't be surprised. The ageing Colonel is particularly embittered and voices the wish that he had continued to fight the war to its conclusion. His 17 sons (all by different mothers who each spent a single night with the famous war hero) are hunted down and killed by the authorities in the space of a week. Things are bad in Macondo and about to get worse. The poorly paid workers of the banana company declare a strike and the fruit rots on the trees. The 120-car train remains idle on the sidings with no bananas to take out. Martial law is declared and the army moves in. Skirmishes break out when they try to take over the work. A crowd gathers to wait for the arrival of a minister in an open space opposite the station. They are ordered to disperse by an officer, but are unwilling (and unable) to do so. The soldiers fire on them with machine guns and thousands are killed. The bodies are removed on the banana train and the Government subsequently denies that the massacre ever took place. Again, we are familiar, from recent South American history, with official mass murder, disappearance and denial.

As if to wash away the bloodstains the massacre is followed by the rains. It rains for four years, eleven months and two days. The whole town becomes a swamp. Aureliano Segundo spends a lot of time obsessively digging ditches looking for the gold that was hidden years ago by a visitor to the house. Úrsula knows where it is but she is not telling. When the rains finally stop the town is in ruins. The banana company has withdrawn and the economy is devastated also. Aureliano Segundo manages to provide for the family with a series of ingenious lotteries. It is not clear how anyone else makes enough money to buy the tickets.

The end of Macondo and a hundred years of solitude

Nevertheless, life in Macondo continues and you will be able to read about the lives of a fifth and sixth generation of Buendías. I will just tell you that Aureliano Segundo fathers three children (the fifth generation) of whom the youngest is a lively and enterprising woman called Amaranta Úrsula. She has the benefit of a European education and comes back with a Belgian husband called Gaston. However, he is frequently away and Amaranta Úrsula becomes increasingly friendly with a young Aureliano who is her nephew. Yes, it's another aunt-and-nephew love affair, and naturally they have the same names. Now we are rapidly approaching the end of the story, and this youngest Aureliano plays a key role in the *dénouement*.

For he is the boy who was taught to read and to take an interest in the parchments by his great-uncle, José Arcadio Segundo. Every morning Aureliano continues his uncle's work. He also has a girlfriend called Nigromanta, who teaches him the arts of love in the afternoons. It's so good to know that he is not a complete workaholic. One day, he is visited by the ghost of Melquíades the gypsy, who confirms that the language of the parchments is Sanskrit.

After a while, Aureliano finds that his passion for Amaranta Úrsula is becoming irresistible. They become lovers and have a child, whom they decide to call Aureliano. Naturally he is born with the tail of a pig but his proud parents are not in the least bothered. We have now reached the last few pages and things begin to go seriously banana shaped. I have decided not to give the ending away. No, it's useless to argue, my mind is made up. All I will tell you is that, as his personal happiness turns to dust, Aureliano finally realises that the writing on the parchment is not just in Sanskrit but in a code which he is suddenly able to understand with complete clarity. This is because a hundred years have passed since the writing began and the time has come for it to reveal itself. You may also have noticed that a powerful wind is getting up and the house is beginning to shake. Aureliano reads on as fast as he can, while with beating hearts and a cold sweat on our brows, we too race through the last few pages. Then we finish in disbelief and read the last chapter again.

In conclusion

When you have recovered, I suggest you read the whole book again and pick up on some of the delights and insights that you missed first time round. This book is so full of riches. It might be seen as a surreal history of South America, a coded political treatise, a family chronicle, a mythological saga, an exploration of the author's unconscious, a tale of obsessive men and determined women or a tragic story of what happens when people lose touch with their feelings and stop communicating. If I haven't already said so, I should add that the writing is breathtakingly brilliant with many vivid phrases that you will remember if you ever find yourself facing the firing squad. And did I mention that it's also very funny?

The text

One Hundred Years of Solitude is available in a paperback edition from Penguin Books, translated from the Spanish by Gregory Rabassa. Extracts from *One Hundred Years of Solitude* by Gabriel García Márquez published by Jonathan Cape. Used by permission of the Random House Group Limited.

Index

646-298-7633